What people are saying abo

"Finally—a book that spells out what so many in the healthcare field have been thinking and wanting for years! HEALTH FOR US ALL provides a highly practical, essential health reform plan for our country. As a clinical psychologist who is very solution-oriented, I'm excited that Dr. Mary Zennett has so expertly and intelligently outlined a comprehensive health plan proposal that emphasizes prevention and wellness, not just treatment of illness and symptoms. In this innovative, inspiring, and workable model, conventional treatment can easily be combined with effective complementary and alternative methods, which will be more cost-effective for everyone concerned. The wealth of information packed into *Health for Us All* helps all caring and responsible practitioners with their patients and clients. It's difficult to find words which adequately describe how passionately I feel about the contents of this book. This is an absolute must-read!"—*Shoshana Bennett, Ph.D., author, Postpartum Depression for Dummies, and internationally renowned speaker and trainer, ClearSky-Inc.com*

"Mary Z has written a tremendously important book. She outlines in great detail the many failures of our current healthcare system. From here she goes to highlight the broad benefits of complementary and alternative medicine both in clinical and economic terms. She correctly advocates CAM as a big part of the solution to our current national healthcare mess. Dr. Z shares her considerable wisdom and insight to bring us closer to a truly comprehensive model of healthcare that will benefit all Americans. Everyone concerned with the creation of healthcare system that cares for health should read this book."—*Scott Shannon, M.D., assistant clinical professor, University of Colorado; department of child psychiatry, Children's Hospital, Denver; director of the first university-based integrative child psychiatry clinic in the United States; founding member of the American Holistic Medical Association, www.wholeness.com*

"Dr. Mary is a passionate leader of health reform. Her book is filled with information that will transform our fractured healthcare system from disease to wellness...get informed on how you can help yourself. The life you save may be your own. Thanks, Doc!"—*Cynthia Brian, the Oprah of the Airwaves; Starstyle—Be the Star You Are!; www. cynthiabrian.com.*

"I...am impressed by your mission to affect real changes in the American healthcare system and by your activism to get that accomplished. I even think you should be part of a task force with the new administration to bring meaningful changes about; they will need people like you who are knowledgeable on the provider side and compassionate enough to be rooted in the patient side as well."—*Britt Mittemeijer; http://www.EasyHealthAndWellness.com; blog: http://www.easy healthandwellness.blogspot.com*

HEALTH FOR US ALL

HEALTH FOR US ALL
The Transformation of U.S. Healthcare

Dr. Mary Zennett

Third Day Press, LLC
Colorado Springs, Colorado

First printing 2009

ISBN 978-0-9818764-3-6

LCCN 2008905667

ATTENTION CORPORATIONS, UNIVERSITIES, COLLEGES, AND PROFESSIONAL ORGANIZATIONS: Quantity discounts are available on bulk purchases of this book for educational, gift purposes, or as premiums for increasing magazine subscriptions or renewals. Special books or book excerpts can also be created to fit specific needs. For information, please contact Third Day Press, LLC; PO Box 75862, Colorado Springs, CO 80970; 1-800-637-4065; www.HealthforUSAll.com; thirddaypress@gmail.com.

*To the good health and well-being of
all United States citizens*

HEALTH FOR US ALL
The Transformation of U.S. Healthcare

Table of Contents

Preface

As a healthcare provider for more than twenty years, I understand well why the time has come to think about a new healthcare system.

The principles of health transformation are actually simple, but they remain formidable because of the large-scale implementation needed. The purpose of this book is to educate and offer potential solutions that represent a complete overhaul of the existing healthcare system, based on core-level principles and values.

I graduated from a large, reputable Midwestern medical school and completed my adult psychiatry training and child/adolescent fellowship at equally well-regarded institutions. I've had my own thriving private practice for years and also have worked in large community mental health centers.

I've cared for patients and families from all walks of life—from families very concerned about their children with ADD, bipolar disorder, and autism, to the chronically mentally ill, the homeless, and the chemically dependent. I've treated many active-duty soldiers, veterans, and their families.

In the late 1990s I became so disheartened with the system that governed the practice of medicine that I completed a two-year curriculum for physicians and earned an executive MBA. This rigorous training taught me not to be afraid of the system but to evaluate the seeming complexities and components critically and strategically. I drew on those skills frequently while formulating recommendations that I believe will lead to health transformation in the upcoming decade.

The primary purpose of any healthcare delivery system is to promote the health and well-being of the people for which it cares. Our current disease-focused industry requires a large-scale transformation that places people first, promotes the quality of their lives, and is proactive about their health from before birth to their last days.

In reality, the current U.S. health-delivery system is so complex, so bureaucratic, and so cumbersome that the patient has been lost in the equation. In their quest for health, people are caught between the two worlds of medicine: conventional medicine and complementary medicine. This book is dedicated to accelerating the integration of these two worlds of healthcare into a system I call *transformational health.* Indeed, this process has been initiated, but progress is slow. Certainly, for patients who access healthcare in both models, this integration cannot come fast enough.

A transformational health-delivery system prevents illness in the first place; such a system is built on relationships, research, individualized care, and most important, hope. It seeks input from the people it serves and from the health practitioners who partner with their patients on lifelong journeys of health and healing. Transformational health integrates the best of both worlds of medicine, empowers people to get healthy and stay healthy, and operates efficiently and cost-effectively. It is a system where principles come before paperwork and people are of far greater value than profits.

In this book, I propose a plan for the integration of conventional and complementary and alternative medicine, as well as changes—some dramatic—to the conventional system. The goal is to create a new health system—one that is much more efficient, streamlined, and focused on long-term health and quality of life for all Americans.

I want to make the principles of health transformation understandable so every citizen—including legislators responsible for decision making—embraces them. Such a model empowers citizens, health providers, and allied health professionals to think and act proactively in advocating and crafting health-transformation efforts.

This call to action will stretch each of us outside of our comfort zone, but it is a necessary process of any transformational effort. In reality, with the national projections for healthcare costs rising in the next ten years, we do not have any other choice. The only alternative is to sit passively and watch our federal budget go bankrupt, and quite frankly, as Americans, this cannot be an option.

The prospect of a healthy America truly affords hope for all. Besides greatly enhancing quality of life and national productivity, establishing a global model of health will set an example for other countries who, like us, are struggling with skyrocketing health costs and escalating rates of chronic illness.

Along with writing this book, I recently founded the National Alliance for Health Reform. The purpose of this organization is to educate citizens and those responsible for decision making in healthcare, and to provide a forum to exchange ideas and help craft public health policies in the twenty-first century.

I thank each of you for your active participation in this transformation of health!

Best wishes,
Dr. Mary Zennett

Acknowledgments

Dr. Chuck Pierce and staff (www.gloryofzion.org), for timeless guidance and inspiration

Sherry Watson, for her tireless grassroots advocacy for the disabled

CEO Space, for years of mentoring and collaboration

Steve Harrison and Quantum Leap for tremendous insights

Sue Collier and her remarkable staff at Self-Publishing Resources

My patients and dedicated staff, who inspire and teach me daily

Nick, for encouragement and expert technical support

Michael, for believing this project will make a positive difference in America

Introduction

AS EVIDENCED IN THE 2008 PRESIDENTIAL ELECTION, healthcare is at the top of the national agenda. Michael Moore's 2007 documentary *Sicko* raised the public's awareness of the more than forty-five million uninsured Americans. Heated debates have only begun to examine the pros and cons of private health insurance and single-payer health coverage.

But a deeper crisis is looming in healthcare, one that is rarely articulated in public debates or by the media in relation to health reform. This crisis stems from the fact that the U.S. healthcare system focuses almost exclusively on treating disease rather than preventing illness. Yet the opportunity that emerges from this crisis is likely to provide a cornerstone of health reform, cost-efficiency, and greatly enhanced quality of life. What we will discuss here impacts every American, from infants to the elderly and the disabled, from the most affluent to the poorest citizens in our country.

The current U.S. healthcare system with its billions of dollars spent on health regulations, paperwork, and financing is really only "half" of a system. These expenditures represent more than 15 percent of the U.S. gross domestic product[1] and are predicted to reach 20 percent before long.[2] How could this possibly represent *half a system*? There are two reasons.

First, two distinct worlds of healthcare currently exist in the United States: The first is the conventional heathcare system, consisting primarily of medications and surgery. When we hear about healthcare reform, this conventional healthcare system is to what people refer. But the other world of medicine is complementary and alternative medicine (CAM). What is CAM? "CAM is a group of diverse medical and healthcare systems, practices, and products that are not presently considered to be part of conventional medicine."[3] CAM therapies include chiropractic, acupuncture, massage, herbs, nutritional, and mind-body therapies, among others. "...[T]he major CAM systems have many common characteristics including a focus on individualizing treatments, treating the whole person, promoting self-care and self-healing, and recognizing the spiritual nature of each individual."[4]

Although CAM is rarely referenced in terms of U.S. health reform, its methods are rising rapidly in popularity and account for billions of dollars per year in annual expenditures.[5] The Centers for Disease Control and Prevention estimated that the U.S. public spent between $36 billion and $47 billion on CAM therapies in 1997.[6] That was more than the U.S. public paid for all hospitalizations that year and approximately one-half of the amount we paid for all out-of-pocket physician services.

The second reason we can consider conventional medicine as only half a system is because the conventional healthcare system is based on treating diseases, primarily with medications and surgeries. The current U.S. healthcare system places virtually no emphasis on wellness and prevention of disease.

Conventional and CAM health systems are huge in their own rights, but what is most disturbing is the nearly total lack of communication between these two systems of healthcare. In many, if not most, conventional settings, integrating nutrition and preventative care is virtually not done. CAM settings, likewise, tend to be very "antidrug" and defensive toward conventional practice. Very little communication and collaboration around patient care exists among practitioners in these systems.

Conventional doctors, often rightfully, speak to the lack of scientific evidence validating CAM modalities. CAM practitioners, also rightfully, point to the potential risks of conventional procedures and medications, surgeries, chemotherapy, radiation, and the like.

The patient is caught between these two worlds, a fact illustrated in chapter 1 of this book. Informed patients stay abreast of new CAM advances largely through word of mouth and the Internet. There is a rise in public awareness that the "feel ill, take a pill" philosophy is not enough. Many in the United States use employer health plans and visit primary-care doctors and also use CAM on a regular basis.

These worlds need to merge for the benefit of the patient. This transformational model of healthcare integrates health and wellness into mainstream conventional health care. It encourages conventional doctors to offer quality health and wellness to patients who are cared for with medications and surgeries in conventional healthcare. This model is driven by the premise that medications and surgeries have a role and a place. Though not all people need medications or surgery, everyone needs health and wellness. We need guidance on quality health and wellness strategies, and those who need medications or surgeries can use wellness principles to get well and stay well. Yes, even people who need medication can be well.

How will integrating CAM into mainstream medicine affect healthcare costs that have already spiraled out of control? Clearly careful study and analysis are in order, but it is rightfully assumed that keeping a population healthy reduces the use of high-priced technologies and surgeries and lowers overall healthcare costs and usage, possibly exponentially. Keeping people well, besides greatly enhancing quality of life, improves productivity by reducing absenteeism, rates of disability, and unemployment.

In March 2002, the White House Commission on Complementary and Alternative Medicine Policy submitted a report containing "legislative and administrative recommendations that would help public policy maximize potential benefits, to consumers and American healthcare, of complementary and alternative medicine (CAM) therapies..."[7] As long as legislators and the U.S. healthcare system follow the policy recommendations in this document, CAM modalities will be researched and available to the public in the next few years.

Can we, as a nation, afford *not* to study the benefits of integrating CAM into our conventional healthcare system?

CHAPTER 1

Patient Impact: Case Studies

Note: The following case studies were compiled through numerous patient histories. To preserve the identities of individuals, the names used do not represent the names of actual patients. The clinical situations, however, occurred in real life.

WHY DOESN'T THE U.S. HEALTHCARE SYSTEM focus on the total health and well-being of all Americans?

In their quest for health, some patients can become caught between the two worlds of medicine with poor results. Consider the two case studies below of Joan and Don. Each has a different outcome, but both illustrate the problems facing patients when they are caught between the two systems.

Joan

Joan was a fifty-five-year-old wife, mother of three, and grandmother of two when she died after a valiant five-year battle with a severe form of breast cancer. What was most tragic is that the cause of her death was not cancer but a fatal heart attack. Joan's death was swift and shocking to the many friends and family who knew and loved her dearly.

When Joan was diagnosed with breast cancer in 1998, she did everything her physicians asked her to do. Her cancer was fairly advanced when she was diagnosed, and her doctors recommended aggressive forms of chemotherapy and radiation. Joan complied with these recommendations and had a bilateral mastectomy as well.

In addition, she had heard from other patients about nutritional supplements that could help offset side effects of chemo and radiation. Joan began taking the nutritional supplements. She had spoken to her doctors about them, and although her doctors were skeptical of the supplements' benefits after learning they were food based and reviewing their high safety record, her doctors didn't see a problem with taking them. She seemed to be recovering well. She had completed two rounds of chemo and a round of radiation, maintaining excellent color and having energy to visit family and friends.

Three months before her death, Joan began taking Lipitor, a commonly prescribed medicine designed to lower cholesterol. Joan suffered from what were likely side effects of Lipitor. Subsequently, with high stress and anxiety levels, she succumbed to a fatal heart attack.

Statins, the class of commonly prescribed cholesterol-lowering medicines to which Lipitor belongs, have muscle spasms and pain as potential side effects. In Joan's case, her legs cramped, causing her quite a bit of pain, and her calf muscles were stiff and spasmed frequently. Her muscles deteriorated, and at times, the pain was agonizing. She lost her sense of balance, which made walking more than a few steps at a time difficult. Already frail from chemotherapy and radiation, she found her symptoms were as devastating emotionally as they were physically. She had worked hard to beat the cancer that was ravaging her body. She was exhausted, physically and mentally, and several months after starting the Lipitor, she died of a heart attack.

Her doctors were amazed to discover she was cancer free when she died. When she was diagnosed, Joan was given a less than 10 percent chance to survive the cancer; no one thought it would have been eradicated from her body. Many, including some of her doctors, believe that without the natural supplements, she never would have beaten the cancer. In the doctors' best estimate, advanced forms of cancer like these rarely go into remission; the goal of treatment is largely to prevent further spread.

Did Joan's battle with cancer make her more susceptible to Lipitor's side effects? Although we will never know for sure, it is a plausible hypothesis. Was Joan too physically and emotionally depleted from the lengthy chemo and radiation to even be a candidate for Lipitor, or any other medication for that matter? Might she have benefited instead from a CAM approach to build up her immune system and support cellular health before any other conventional treatments were rendered?

There are many stories like Joan's. Consider thirty-five-year-old Don from California, who was diagnosed with multiple sclerosis (MS) twelve years ago. He had been an award-winning athlete in high school, primarily excelling in basketball. He attended college on a full athletic scholarship until MS hit.

Don

Don's physical decline came hard and fast. He had maintained an incredible spirit and coped well when faced with life's pressures, and when he became afflicted with MS, he used this same spirit and positive attitude. But his illness precluded him from vigorous exercise—previously one of his best coping strategies.

Friends led him to a doctor who helped him embark on a process of cleansing and detoxification. He had heard about several nutritional supplements from an MS support group. And although no products can claim to cure, treat, or mitigate disease, he found the benefits of both classes of supplements remarkable.

His doctor believed that his claims about the supplements were unfounded and felt Don was already receiving similar ingredients in other nutritional drinks he was taking. Confused, Don stopped both sets of supplements but continued the nutritional drink. Within a month, his condition deteriorated. He is currently confined to a wheelchair, worn out, and depressed.

Did Don's belief in the two sets of supplements contribute to his recovery? Perhaps. Did the supplements contain ingredients that were helpful to his recovery on a cellular level? Probably.

With his friends, he had been ecstatic about the prospects of health and healing. It is not clear if he shared the same enthusiasm with his healthcare provider.

Currently, many patients who use CAM therapies do not share this information with their conventional doctor. In a study published in the *New England Journal of Medicine*, 72 percent of respondents did not inform their medical doctor of their use of unconventional therapy.[8]

In a study by Winslow and Shapiro, 751 physicians in Denver, Colorado, were asked about their experience with CAM and how they talked to their patients about CAM. Seventy-six percent of the doctors reported using CAM with their patients but "Few physicians felt comfortable discussing CAM with their patients," and the "overwhelming majority (84 %) thought they needed to learn more about CAM to adequately address patient concerns."[9]

Clearly, the need to study the safety, efficacy, and appropriateness of CAM approaches is a vital component of any health transformation efforts.

Mr. Smith

Now consider Mr. Smith, a fifty-five-year-old gentleman with diabetes, high blood pressure, and obesity. He currently takes three medications to lower his blood pressure and two medications to help control his blood sugar. His daughter, a certified nutritionist, has worked hard with him to establish a healthier diet, which includes taking nutritional supplements. In addition, she accompanies him on a walk three times per week.

Mr. Smith has a wonderful relationship with his daughter and a good working relationship with his doctor. He didn't feel comfortable telling his doctor that he was taking extra nutritional supplements for fear of what his doctor would think. So instead of explaining his entire regimen, including the diet and exercise, Mr. Smith didn't discuss any of it with his doctor. He also didn't want to hurt his daughter's feelings by getting into a conflict with his doctor and risk stopping the supplements.

After three months on the diet, exercise, and supplement regimen, Mr. Smith experienced a sudden blood pressure drop and fell down a flight of stairs at home. He suffered a leg fracture but fortunately, no other problems.

When he told his doctor what had happened, his blood pressure and blood sugar were so improved that his doctor reduced his blood pressure medications to one and lowered his blood sugar medication dosages. His doctor agreed to monitor him closely, knowing that these healthy lifestyle changes made it more likely he would be able to lower his patient's dosages even further and possibly discontinue some medication.

Fortunately, Mr. Smith and his doctor had a genuine respect for each other. The doctor assured Mr. Smith that he wanted to hear about any and all lifestyle changes in the future. Mr. Smith was relieved.

This is the outcome for which all patients should strive.

CHAPTER 2

Understanding Our Conventional HealthCare System

THE TRANSFORMATION OF HEALTHCARE needs to begin in the minds and hearts of every American because health affects us all. But before we evaluate models of integration and transformation in healthcare, we will examine the current conventional healthcare system in the United States.

In 2003, healthcare represented 15.2 percent of the gross national product (GNP), and that figure rises annually.[10] According to the Centers for Medicare and Medicaid Services (CMS), the United States was projected to spend over $2.2 trillion on healthcare in 2007, or just under $7,500 per U.S. resident.[11] According to the CMS, by 2016, "healthcare spending in the United States is projected to reach just over $4.1 trillion and comprise 19.6 percent of GDP."[12]

"One in every six Americans under the age of 65 did not have health insurance (18%) in 2006, for a total of 46.5 million people."[13] Between 2000 and 2004, the number of uninsured grew by nearly 6 million, and between 2004 and 2006, an additional 3.4 million U.S. citizens were uninsured.[14]

People from all walks of life lack health insurance. Any small-business owner knows the dilemma of providing health insurance for him- or herself as well as employees. The skyrocketing costs of premiums have forced many small-business owners to not offer employees any health insurance and have forced still others out of business altogether. Young people entering the workforce are another subgroup in the U.S. population that often lacks health insurance. Often in school and working part-time, they do not qualify for health insurance or cannot afford the premiums. Many single moms lack health insurance, although their children often qualify for state subsidized programs. An increasing number of adults in their forties and fifties are also uninsured. Either a layoff or illness has prevented them from maintaining full-time employment, and because they often are afflicted with a chronic health challenge, the downward spiral takes its course. An alarming number of U.S. adults in this position find themselves bankrupt, homeless, and unable to afford the healthcare they need. Indeed, more than eight in ten uninsured citizens come from working families.

Many healthcare professionals agree that lack of access to care is among the greatest strains on our healthcare system today. This includes care for people covered partly or minimally under health insurance. My staff and I spend almost as much time being creative in helping people get the care they need as we do treating patients. This is no small statement, as we care for large numbers of patients daily. And we are not alone. I hear stories daily of healthcare staff providing free care, markedly reduced care, writing off copayments and insurance deductibles, providing pharmaceutical samples, helping patients apply for patient assistance programs from pharmaceutical companies, or offering patients taxi vouchers just to get home from doctors visits. Such activities have become an additional and standard part of a health provider's already very busy day.

Here in the United States, with the highest per capita costs on healthcare in the world and where costs are rising exponentially, the World Health Organization ranks the overall quality of our healthcare system as thirty-seventh.[15]

How the system evolved

To understand the evolution of our current health-delivery system, we need to go back to the early 1900s. Melissa Thomasson presents an excellent historical perspective in "Health Insurance in the United States." According to Thomasson, "Given the rudimentary state of medical technology before 1920, most people had very low medical expenditures.... In fact, the chief cost associated with illness was not the cost of medical care, but rather the fact that 'sick people couldn't work and did not get paid.'"[16] Even then, people had the option to purchase "sickness" insurance—similar to disability insurance today—to replace lost wages in the event of illness.

Physician licensing and costs of medical technology contributed to rising health costs in the early 1900s. First, the American Medical Association (AMA) established licensing standards and stringent requirements for physicians in order to treat patients. Second, "Advances in medical technology, along with the growing acceptance of medicine as a science, led to the development of hospitals as treatment centers and helped to encourage sick people to visit physicians and hospitals."[17] Before this time, people were treated in their homes, and if someone got sick, there was little hope for recovery.

Thomasson quoted Charles E. Rosenberg in "The Care of Strangers," who stated, "By the 1920s...prospective patients were influenced not only by the hope of healing, but by the image of a new kind of medicine—precise, scientific and effective."[18] Thomasson continues, "This scientific aura began to develop in part as licensure and standards of care among practitioners increased, which led to an increase in the cost of providing medical care."[19]

By 1932, the American Hospital Association encouraged the development of prepaid health insurance. By then, people sought care in hospitals, but after the Great Depression, they had difficulty paying for their medical care. Health insurance was borne in an effort to create a system that would meet the needs of all people and ensure that the hospital bills were paid. But Thomasson points out, "The prepayment plan also clearly benefited hospitals by providing them with a way to earn income during a time of failing hospital revenue."[20]

Although the desire to meet people's needs was a noble one, fiscal accountability or oversight in regard to medical expenditures was lacking, even then. "Medical insurance does not just pay for medical care—it shapes the medical care delivery systems, determines what treatments are developed, and formulates our view of what constitutes medical care."[21] In the earliest days of medical insurance, it was unclear who determined what treatments were paid for or why, and this is a major problem in today's system.

In the NYU Annual Survey of American Law, Thomas R. McLean and Edward P. Richards quoted George D. Lundberg and James Stacy in regard to the development of the first Blue Cross plan in 1929: "At first, the purpose of this type of plan was not so much to provide health benefits as to keep cash flowing into hospitals."[22] And in Thomasson's words, "Commercial insurance companies were reluctant to even offer health insurance early in the century...they feared that offering health insurance would not be profitable."[23] To minimize risks of adverse selection that could come with insuring the sick and unemployed, Blue Cross and Blue Shield, the first to enter the health insurance market, chose to insure only young and healthy workers.

Fiscal problems really exploded in the sixties with the development of high-priced technological advances, such as cardiac bypass surgery, organ transplant, and chemotherapy. In earlier years, insurance had paid for interventions such as antibiotic treatment and occasional surgical procedures. In the 1960s and 1970s, insurance plans liberally paid doctor bills, hospital bills, and bills for procedures and equipment (such as X-rays and electrocardiograms). They also were generous with payments for prescriptions. Annual health costs rose so exorbitantly during the 1980s and 1990s, managed-care organizations moved to the forefront of medical care to closely monitor and contain medical costs. Managed care is "a general term for organizing doctors, hospitals and other providers into groups, in order to enhance the quality and cost-effectiveness of health care."[24]

While practicing medicine in the early 1990s, I distinctly remember wondering "who turned the treadmill on high speed?" Almost overnight daily practice, with the advent of managed care, felt like running a marathon, with caring for patients the worthwhile part of the day. The rest of the day was spent on high speed, processing paperwork, answering phone calls from insurance and managed-care companies, and from patients anxious that their health bill was going to be denied by insurance or managed care, calling for prior authorization for prescriptions or any special testing ordered. I've said many times, we've learned to take care of our paperwork very well; I hope we've done as good a job of actually caring for our patients.

Certainly, the past few years in medicine have brought an array of new pharmaceutical products, along with advertisements and now commercials promoting lawsuits against pharmaceutical companies.

HMOs develop

One component of managed care includes heath maintenance organizations (HMOs). HMOs, a form of health insurance, were designed to offer comprehensive health coverage for both hospital and physician services. HMOs were also intended to focus on preventative health. They were to promote wellness, offering hope that with sound preventative care, people would not need expensive high-tech diagnostic tests and procedures. Hence, hospital stays—a very high-ticket item in any healthcare budget—would be reduced.

The concept of preventative care was a great one. However, the preventative services HMO plans offered were typically routine screenings—mammograms, pelvic exams, blood pressure exams, and prostate screenings for early detection of disease. They also offered some programs for weight reduction, lowering cholesterol, and managing high blood pressure. These services were not designed to prevent illness but to detect illnesses that had already developed. So how did these preventative services enhance quality of life and cut healthcare costs?

Managed care organizations adopted "utilization review." Utilization refers to "use of services. Utilization is commonly examined in terms of patterns or rates of use of...service such as hospital care, physician visits, prescription drugs."[25] This meant the HMO, in this case, had "utilization standards" of what services would or would not be covered. Certain prescriptions were approved and adopted in the HMO formulary, and others denied. The HMO could hire specialists to review the care that was being administered. Emphasis was placed on the efficiency of the delivery of the care—in other words, how few sessions were needed to achieve a desired patient outcome.

The utilization review process is incredibly time consuming for a physician as well as the staff a doctor needs to manage the paperwork and the process. Because the HMOs had cut doctors' fees so substantially, lack of revenue precluded them from hiring the number of qualified people necessary to process claims, organize the authorization paperwork for the doctor to complete additional patient services, and coordinate the physician-to-physician phone call reviews and additional documentation to support ongoing treatment. This level of administrative staff doesn't account for the clinical and receptionist staff necessary to interact with patients and serve their needs. Nor does it account for the time and energy the doctor needs to spend justifying care, taking precious time away from direct patient care.

I can attest to the impact of managed care and utilization review on practitioners and patients. During the advent of managed care in the 1990s, I've mentioned feeling as if someone had turned up the speed on a treadmill, and none of us—not doctors, patients, nurses, or administrative staff—was getting off. The only way to slow down the pace of practice with managed care was to refuse to accept any insurance reimbursement or to leave practice.

I've spoken with many of my patients over the years about their experience in the office while they were waiting for appointments. Many patients have commented how busy and stressed everyone is. Full waiting rooms and little time to visit with doctors, nurses, or receptionists—all this is the result of managed care and utilization review.

Managed care and utilization review are paperwork- and phone-intense and do not relate to the direct care of the patient. But if a doctor's staff did not tend to this paperwork, patient visits would not get approved and insurance claims would be denied. This paperwork consumes valuable time and money, and takes enormous time away from patient care.

Another issue that comes up frequently with patients is the feeling of betrayal when they learn that their insurance company will not pay for certain services, or in other cases, an entire hospital stay. For many patients and family members, affording the insurance premium is no small accomplishment. Most people understand their insurance company has copayments, deductibles, and some service restrictions. But most patients do not even know their insurance reimbursement must be approved by a third-party managed-care company—an agency represented by a person with whom they have never met.

Where we stand today

As we've stated, policyholders believe that because they have insurance coverage they are covered. This used to be true, but now managed-care companies have taken over a lot of authority in determining what healthcare services will or will not be covered.

Managed-care companies were designed to closely monitor care and protect the insurance companies from abuse and fraud. Currently, the restrictions in healthcare are so great that it often seems from a patient and a doctor's perspective that a managed-care company exists to deny care.

A patient could be admitted to a hospital through the emergency room late at night, only to learn the next day that the hospital stay is not covered, and the patient is responsible for the entire bill. The last thing a patient who is physically ill needs is additional financial burden, but unfortunately, this scenario is all too common.

Managed care has all but driven healthcare providers out of medicine. Recent statistics confirm "nearly half of physicians age 50 or older plan to leave medicine within the next three years," and 56 percent of physicians cite managed care as their biggest professional frustration; nearly 50 percent of doctors indicate that managed care was a 'significant factor' or the 'single most significant factor' in their decision to change their style of practice."[26]

Imagine doing a job, documenting the details of the job, and then adding additional layers of paperwork to document the job again. That's what managed care has created. Healthcare professionals bemoan, "When do we get to care for our patients?" Although its intentions were initially good, the managed-care system has evolved into a major web of bureaucracy that takes doctors and their staff away from patient care, forcing them to focus instead on paperwork to obtain authorizations for the care they provide. The strain on patients and health providers from managed care is relentless. It often feels as though the health service offered the patient is denied just as fast as it is rendered.

Critics of managed-care plans, including some consumers, employees, and providers, argue that their practices threaten quality. They contend that most health plans focus primarily on a bottom line of payment, not patient care. This, in turn, means that the health plans deny care that physicians and other caregivers deem necessary. Other critics, including some employers, believe that managed-care plans have not succeeded at controlling costs. According to Kaiser Daily Health Policy Report, "health insurance claims denials cost billions in administrative costs."[27]

Charles V. Burton, MD, a distinguished U.S. neurosurgeon and publisher of more than one hundred peer-reviewed medical papers, scientific papers, books, and *The Burton Report*, found that

a 1990 survey performed by the inspector general of the U.S. Health and Human Services Department, which reviewed 500,000 cataract operations funded by Medicare, demonstrated that the United States government paid $13.3 million for utilization reviewers to save $1.4 million in possibly unnecessary surgical costs. These and other data, made clear that utilization review was simply replacing medical costs with administrative costs."[28]

The unspoken tension and limited time with patients, a hallmark of the managed-care era, also has contributed to increased threats of malpractice lawsuits. A recent study sought to determine why only 6 percent of the nation's obstetricians accounted for 85 percent of the malpractice claim payments. Evidently, the quality of the care did not differ significantly from the quality of the care from doctors who had no malpractice claim. The highest number of claims came from physicians

> who had the highest number of dissatisfied patients. These dissatisfied patients remarked that their doctor spent less than ten minutes on average with them during their visit, ignored their questions and comments, did not keep them adequately informed, and generally showed no concern for their well-being.[29]

Indeed, the "treadmill" of medical practice, where a doctor sees ten to twenty patients in an hour's time, does not offer the time for the physician and patient to even establish rapport, much less provide time for the doctor to listen to the patient's concerns, offer consultation, and suggest some meaningful treatment recommendations.

The finances that sustain this treadmill warrant close scrutiny. *New York Times* columnist Paul Krugman writes, "It is a fact that insurers spend a lot of money looking for ways to reject insurance claims.... Meanwhile, healthcare providers "spend billions on 'denial management', employing specialist firms...to fight the insurers."[30]

In my large and busy private practice, the advent of managed care required hiring a team of specialists to process the volumes of paperwork claims and manage the insurance denial letters. It was no small feat to collect enough revenue to pay for the quality specialists and keep my clinic lights on. I can recall asking myself many times, "What happened to the focus on patient care?"

Krugman concludes that the larger problem of the U.S. healthcare system "isn't the behavior of any individual company. It's the ugly incentives provided by a system in which giving care is punished, while denying it is rewarded."[31]

And where does complementary and alternative medicine (CAM) fit in with managed care?

It doesn't. In most cases, CAM is not a covered benefit. So people who want to be proactive and prevent illness in the first place currently have little to no support from their insurance or managed-care company.

The entire conventional healthcare system is largely focused on accurate diagnosis and treatment, which mainly consists of medications or surgeries. To date, little preventative care exists in our current conventional healthcare system. True preemptive care goes beyond the early detection of disease. It is a way of life that encompasses learning and mastering good health habits. The principles of CAM encompass preventative healthcare, and conventional medicine's strengths lie in being able to treat diseases. For us to fully enjoy health and contain costs, both worlds of healthcare need to be integrated.

How gratifying it would be to participate in a healthcare system that helps people get and stay healthy, and prevent the pain and suffering of chronic illness, and that will be there if a person does get sick. That's what a transformed healthcare system looks like—and we are so ready for it here in America.

Conclusion

Conventional healthcare has evolved over the years and is very expensive, yet it does not adequately meet the comprehensive healthcare needs of U.S. citizens. With its efforts focused on containing costs, managed care has actually caused more waste and hindered the patient-doctor relationship.

Conventional medicine does not currently focus on prevention. Preventative care as it currently exists in conventional healthcare is usually defined as discovering the early states of a disease, rather than actually preventing the disease.

People need a system that truly focuses on prevention as well as treatment in accordance with the Hippocratic Oath.

CHAPTER 3

The Plight of the Uninsured

IT IS NO SECRET THAT 46.5 MILLION Americans currently lack health insurance, and those numbers are rising. In 2006, one in every six Americans was uninsured, constituting 18 percent of the population.[32]

Who are the uninsured?

A recent monograph published by the Kaiser Family Foundation in October 2007, "The Uninsured," identifies just who these people are:

> More than eight in ten uninsured come from working families. Employer-sponsored insurance is not an option for most uninsured employees—for 70 percent of them, their employer or their spouse's employer do not offer health benefits, or they are not eligible for benefits.[33]

Some employees are not eligible for employer-sponsored insurance because they are part-time employees, recent hires, or employees who chose not to enroll because of the high cost of their portion of the payment. About one-fifth of the uninsured report being contacted by a collection agency about unpaid medical bills in the last year; about one-third report spending less on basic needs such as food and heat to pay medical bills.

I talk to health providers daily who agree that caring for the uninsured is one of the top priorities in any health-reform efforts. Today, emergency rooms and community clinics provide much of the care for uninsured patients. Doctors, nurses, and allied health professionals do an amazing job but the work is wearying for all. Most clinics are acutely understaffed to meet the needs of the large numbers of people who desperately need the care.

Amy Davidoff, PhD, and Genevieve M. Kenney, PhD, researchers commissioned by the Robert Wood Johnson Foundation to report prevalence and impact of chronic health challenges in the uninsured, reported that almost half of uninsured adults with chronic conditions "forgo needed medical care and prescription drugs at much higher rates than their insured counterparts."[34]

The consequences

What are the consequences of forgoing or delaying medical care?

In "Care Without Coverage, Too Little, Too Late" by the Institute of Medicine (IOM), "One national study found that, over a 17-year follow-up period, adults who lacked health insurance at the outset had a 25 percent greater chance of dying than did those who have private health insurance."[35]

The main findings of this report issued by the Institute's Committee on the Consequences of Uninsurance include
> working-age Americans without health insurance are more likely to receive too little medical care and receive it too late; be sicker and die sooner; receive poorer care when they are in the hospital, even for acute situations like a motor vehicle crash.[36]

The IOM report concludes "the best health outcomes are possible only if the uninsured obtain coverage before the onset of any illness or injury,"[37] speaking clearly to the need for preventative and early intervention care.

Tragically, most health practitioners today report seeing patients who are "sicker and sicker." In part, this relates to people waiting so late—and in many cases too late—to seek care and have their health restored.

In "Why Insurance Matters," Families USA points to deaths of eighteen thousand Americans between the ages of twenty-five and sixty-four because of lack of insurance. "This makes uninsurance the sixth leading cause of death, ahead of HIV/AIDS and diabetes."[38] IOM confirms that

the poorer health status of uninsured adults at the time of hospitalization is compounded by their experiences as inpatients. They receiver fewer needed services, worse quality care, and have a greater risk of dying in the hospital or shortly after discharge.[39]

We treat patients who have not had lab tests or routine preventative tests in more than twenty years. And it is true; when they receive the same quality inpatient treatment, their physical condition is so depleted, their immune system so compromised, they, as a group, do not fare as well in terms of disease recovery upon discharge. And how can they? Many live in their cars, in shelters, in the mountains, under bridges. Even the working uninsured tend to have much lower rates of recovery than those with good access to healthcare and prevention screenings.

The number of young adults without insurance is increasing, with young adults between the ages of nineteen and twenty-nine representing the "fastest growing segment of the population without health insurance."[40] According to Commonwealth Fund senior program officer Sara Collins, "Policy changes such as increasing the age of eligibility for public programs and continued parental coverage would stabilize insurance among young adults and ease their transition to adulthood."[41]

The Kaiser Commission on Medicaid and the Uninsured concludes:

A conservative estimate based on the full range of studies is that a reduction in mortality of 5–15% could be expected if the uninsured were to gain continuous health coverage.... Better health would improve annual earnings by about 10–30 percent and would increase educational attainment." [42]

This underscores how essential good health is to the quality of life and productivity of individuals—and our nation as a whole. With good health, virtually everything is

CHAPTER 4

Why Are Health Costs So High?

THE UNITED STATES SPENDS THE LARGEST amount of money per capita in the world on the healthcare of its citizens, with spending growing at the fastest rate worldwide.[43] All efforts at health transformation must include a careful analysis of the complex reasons for these skyrocketing costs.

The sources of exorbitant U.S. healthcare costs fall into two major categories: (1) increasing rates of chronic illness in the United States, and (2) excess spending in the existing U.S. healthcare system

Let's begin by examining sources of excess spending in the current healthcare system.

Excessive spending in the current system

Let's look carefully at why so much money is spent in the current U.S. healthcare system. Tracking the excessive costs leads us first to medical technology and then to regulation.

Medical technology

A great deal of analysis has been done over the years on U.S. healthcare costs, including an excellent summary by the Kaiser Family Foundation. The March 2007 study revealed that "healthcare experts point to the development and diffusion of medical technology as primary factors in explaining the persistent difference between health-care spending and overall economic growth, with some arguing that new medical technology may account for about one-half or more of real long-term spending growth."[44] The following summarizes this excellent article:

...the term "medical technology" can be used to refer to the procedures, equipment and processes by which medical care is delivered. Examples...include new medical and surgical procedures (e.g., angioplasty,joint replacements), drugs...medical devices (e.g., CT scanners, implantable defibrillators), and new support systems (e.g., electronic medical records...telemedicine). There is very little in the field of medicine that does not use some type of medical technology and that has not been affected by new technology.[45]

Although examples of miracles through technology abound, the following sobering question exists: Why are so many U.S. citizens still sick? What is the role of low-cost, preventative strategies to minimize the use of high-priced technologies? And in a highly complex, highly regulated industry such as healthcare, who decides that the national health priority agenda will be "prevention first"?

Another must-read for current health-cost analysis is Maggie Mahar's *Money Driven Medicine: The Real Reason Health Care Costs So Much.* Mahar quotes Karen Davis, president of the Commonwealth Fund, who states,

Health care spending in the U.S. is higher because we pay higher prices for the same services; we have higher administrative costs; and we perform more complex, specialized procedures...over the past 25 years power in our health care system has shifted from the physician to the corporation.... A physician pledged to put his patient's interests ahead of his own financial interests. The corporation, by contrast, is legally bound to put its shareholders' interests first. Thus, many decisions about how to allocate health care dollars have become marketing decisions. Drug makers, device makers, and insurers decide which products to develop based not on what patients need but on what their marketers tell them to sell—and produce the highest profit.[46]

Thus, marketing and potential profits currently govern which medications and technologies are researched and which are brought to market. And although technology has its benefits, who decides to research potentially effective, less expensive prevention and wellness strategies?

The use of high-priced technologies is driven by something else: the number of medical school graduates seeking high-priced specialties that use these technologies. Rising medical school tuition and mounting debts appear to be driving students' decisions to pursue specialty medical fields. According to the American Medical Association, "students with high debt are less likely to pursue family practice and primary care specialties."[47] Thus, the market for high-priced technologies appears, in part, to be self-selecting, driven by medical students' choice of specialty.

Professor of history and public health at Columbia University Dr. David Rosner elaborates:

The 1960s saw a critique of medicine that emphasized the maldistribution of physicians, their extraordinary income, and the elitist, conservative nature of the AMA. Further, the dearth of hospital and physicians' services for the nation's poor added an obvious political dimension to the arguments over the medical profession...all these complaints reflected a growing sense that medicine has become far too removed from the population it served and that the sensitivity of medical practice had been sacrificed to the altar of science and technology.[48]

The dilemmas of which products and services are "reasonable and customary" and which are too costly abound in practice today. As a psychiatrist, I do see benefits of newer and safer medications. I recall making rounds in our State Mental Hospital back in the early 1980s, seeing the same highly sedated patients sitting in the same place day after day, month after month. Indeed a fair percentage of patients with severe mental illness do have markedly improved quality of life on the newer antipsychotics. But these medications are not side-effect free and are incredibly expensive. Medications such as Haldol and Thorazine had all but eliminated their hallucinations, but what about their quality of life?

Thus every session with a patient today requires weighing the potential risks and the potential benefits—both short- and long-term—of every medication prescribed. And affordability of these newer medications has become a routine part of the clinical discussion between patient and doctor.

One concern I have is a reactive philosophy of some healthcare cost containment strategies that strongly encourage almost complete use of the older medications with high side-effect risks. The older medications have their place, and indeed certain patients respond well to them. But instead of relying on the older medications to contain healthcare costs, why are we not focusing on adding health and wellness to all patients' medication regimens? Why are we not closely examining the benefits of lowering costs with enhanced quality of life by helping people get healthy and stay healthy? This strategy involves being proactive rather than adopting more reactive strategies to healthcare costs already spiraling out of control.

The role of regulation

Another factor in understanding medical costs is skyrocketing regulatory costs. "The high cost of health services regulation is responsible for more than seven million Americans lacking health insurance."[49] According to University of Rochester health economist Charles Phelps, "The U.S. health care system, while among the most 'market oriented' in the industrialized world, remains the most intensively regulated sector of the U.S. economy."[50]

Christopher J. Conover is assistant research professor with Center for Health Policy, Law and Management at the Terry Sanford Institute of Public Policy at Duke University. Conover presented before the Committee on Health, Education, Labor and Pensions, after careful analysis of the figures, "the net burden of health services regulation likely exceeds the annual cost of covering all 44 million uninsured."[51] He writes,

Students of regulation have known for decades that the burden of regulation on the U.S. economy is sizable...given that the health industry is among the most heavily regulated sectors in the U.S. economy.... Moreover, 4,000 more Americans die every year from costs associated with health insurance regulation (22,000) than from lack of health insurance (18,000)."[52]

Conover concludes: "Finding ways to reduce or eliminate this excess [regulatory] cost should be an urgent priority for policymakers. ...Medical tort reform offers the most promising target for regulatory cost savings, followed by FDA reform, selected access-oriented health insurance regulations (e.g. mandated health benefits), and quality-oriented health facilities regulations (e.g. accreditation and licensure)."[53]

Areas of current health regulation include:
- Health facilities regulation
- Heath professionals regulation
- Health insurance regulation
- FDA regulation of pharmaceuticals and medical devices
- Medical malpractice

To healthcare practitioners, more regulations mean two things: increased paperwork and less time with patients. There is no doubt that some regulation will always be necessary in healthcare, but not at the expense of the purpose of our healthcare system, which is to care for our patients.

Conclusion

The issues of costly medical technology and excess administrative and regulatory costs must be addressed for us, as a nation, to move forward into a new model of healthcare. A new model with the old issues will quickly become our old model—only we will have spent billions shifting models without addressing the roots of the problems.

The issue of profits driving research and health education is a huge one. Citizen education and input is vital; citizens' tax dollars and insurance premiums are funding much of this care. Insurance companies, likewise, can become tremendous advocates of prevention. Would an insurance carrier prefer to spend millions of dollars on high-priced technology or pennies on the dollar for wellness and preventative care? We need to align our incentives if we are to make healthcare a great value again, as we improve the health status of our citizens. Given the strains to the GDP of the costs of U.S. healthcare, these discussions and decisions will be a must, not an option, in days and years to come, and they need to happen sooner rather than later.

We will discuss more about research directives in a transformational healthcare system. One thing is for certain: Research must be patient-centered, including emphasis on health, wellness and prevention. It is estimated that approximately 1 percent of healthcare is dedicated to true wellness and prevention. Let's make it more than 50 percent and greatly lower the incidence of chronic illness in the United States.

Increasing rates of chronic illness

According to a recent report by the Milken Institute, Americans with chronic illnesses cost the U.S. economy more than $1 trillion per year, with this figure predicted to reach $6 trillion by year 2050, unless people take steps to improve their health.[54] The report also indicated that a focus on prevention in U.S. healthcare could save $1.6 trillion by 2023.[55]

According to Ross DeVol, the director of health and regional economics of the Milken Institute and the report's primary author, "More than half of Americans suffer from chronic disease. Every year, millions of people are diagnosed, and every year, millions die of these diseases."[56]

The Milken report identified the seven most common chronic conditions as "cancer, hypertension, mental disorders, heart disease, pulmonary conditions, diabetes, and stroke."[57] It stated that "the human and economic toll of chronic diseases on patients' families and society is enormous" and projected a 42 percent increase in cases of the seven chronic illnesses in 2023 with $4.2 trillion in treatment costs and lost economic productivity.[58]

Many patients in the United States with chronic conditions receive their medical care through Medicare. About 62 percent of Medicare beneficiaries have two or more chronic conditions; 40 percent have three or more. Those with three or more see, on average, ten different physicians during a typical year.[59] Roughly 80 percent of all Medicare dollars are spent for about 20 percent of beneficiaries.[60] And as I discuss later, the only way to lower health costs for patients with multiple, complex, chronic health challenges is through a concerted effort to incorporate prevention and wellness into their daily lives.

Enhanced quality of life is reason enough to embrace wellness and preventative care in the day-to-day practice of medicine. Now with data on skyrocketing healthcare costs of chronic illness, it seems clear that we can no longer afford not to incorporate prevention and wellness into day-to-day healthcare.

Even with all this expenditure, the World Health Organization ranked the current U.S. health system a dismal thirty-seventh. This was particularly striking for women's health issues, with the United States receiving an "unsatisfactory" report card in the first comprehensive assessment of the overall health of women. According to the report, "America's policy makers are letting women down with inadequate, ineffective and inconsistent healthcare policies that too often focus on illness rather than health."[61]

In addition, a recent Kaiser Daily Health Policy Report study compared the health of U.S. and British residents over age fifty-five and ranked the U.S. residents as "much sicker"—with higher rates of diabetes, heart attack, stroke, lung disease, and cancer.[62]

According to epidemiologist and study coauthor, Michael Marmot,

> At every point in the social hierarchy there is more illness in the U.S. than in England and the differences are really quite dramatic. ...Health insurance cannot be the central reason for better health outcomes in England because the top socioeconomic status tier of the U.S. population have close to universal access, but their health outcomes are often worse than those of their English counterparts."[63]

According to Marmot,

The marked disparities were primarily due to...differences in the circumstances in which people live. Work, job insecurity, the nature of communities, residential communities, et cetera.... I think that's the place we should try and look."[64]

Essentially Marmot is speaking of the role of quality of life—or lack of it—in the daily life of U.S. citizens and the health-robbing impact on the lives of Americans. Thus, a plausible contributor to the rise in rates of chronic health challenges in the United States is the decline of quality of life.

Let's examine four factors that directly impact quality of life for Americans and increase the risk of chronic illness: stress, depression, nutritional depletion, and aging.

Stress

According to the American Institute of Stress, stress is America's number-one health problem.[65] Hans Seyle coined the term "fight or flight" to illustrate the response to stress that helped our ancestors survive generations ago.[66] Acute stress prepares us for emergencies, which is why we can mobilize our resources in a crisis. Chronic stress, on the other hand, affects health through complex physiological mechanisms. Chronic stress has been linked to diseases such as heart disease, stomach ailments, hormonal problems, and immune system disorders.

Stress leads to increased heart rate and blood pressure, initially increasing blood flow to the brain to improve focus, concentration, and decision making; stress increases blood sugar initially to provide more fuel for energy in the brain. Stress wreaks havoc on the immune system long-term and is directly linked to autoimmune illnesses such as fibromyalgia, chronic fatigue, and lupus, to name a few. Stress can trigger insulin resistance, which predisposes a person to the onset of diabetes. Tension headaches are highly associated with stress, as well as stomach distress, sleep disturbance, and impairments in focus and concentration.[67]

Many sources of stress appear in modern life. The American Institute of Stress identifies job stress as far and away the leading cause of stress for adults, but stress levels have also escalated in children, teenagers, college students and the elderly for other reasons: increased crime, violence and other threats to personal safety, pernicious peer pressures that lead to substance abuse and other unhealthy lifestyle habits, social isolation and loneliness, the erosion of family and religious values and ties; the loss of other strong sources of social support that are powerful stress busters.[68]

The National Institute for Occupational Safety and Health defined job stress as "the harmful physical and emotional responses that occur when the requests of the job do not match the capabilities, resources or needs of the worker."[69]

Other life stressors include loneliness, relationship problems, and long-term financial stress, which are highly prevalent in our current society. The day-to-day stressors American workers face are many: the role of automation, which causes workers to feel like robots; accelerated paperwork and productivity demands; downsizing; and the need for each worker to perform the tasks of two to three workers.

In addition to the emotional components, job stress is correlated with the following:

- Cardiovascular disease
- Psychological disorders
- Workplace injury
- Suicide
- Cancer
- Ulcers
- Impaired immune function

According to Mary Corbitt Clark, executive director of Winning Workplaces, "Job stress is a key driver of health care costs. According to the Journal of Occupational and Environmental Medicine, healthcare expenditures are nearly 50 percent greater for workers reporting high levels of stress."[70]

The impact of Western society's fast-paced life has only begun to be recognized as taking a toll on the health of Americans. This stress takes a silent but pervasive toll on all of us. First, because we are too busy, moving too fast to take account of what's happening, and even more so, feeling helpless and without options as to what to do. What is the impact of this pace on the mental and emotional health of our youngsters?

Integrating health and wellness in a transformed healthcare model will need to build in time for Americans to live more balanced lives. Again, with the health costs of stress, we as a society must factor in strategies for a more balanced work day—and life—for Americans.

I talk to working parents daily who would love to attend health-related community or church family activities, but by the end of the day are just too tired and too stressed to attend. What toll does this take on the health of the American workforce—the backbone of our economy? It would seem that a proactive response to keeping our workforce healthy—physically, mentally, emotionally—would be the best thing for the U.S. economy today.

Depression

A known correlation exists between stress and the onset of depression. According to the Mayo Foundation for Medical Education and Research, "persistent or chronic stress has the potential to put vulnerable individuals at a substantially increased risk of depression, anxiety and many other emotional difficulties."[71]

Depression is one of the greatest health challenges in America today. One in eighteen people, which constitutes 5.3 percent or 14.4 million people, is treated for depression in the United States each year. Based on lifetime prevalence, depression is as common in the labor market as in the general population.[72] Depression has been linked to many health challenges, including stroke, cancer, dementia, heart disease, and even Parkinson's disease.[73]

Currently, health reform measures do not adequately address this pandemic of depression, and all too often people who need and would benefit from the services are uninsured, marginally insured, or cannot afford the copayments for service on their existing health plans.

Many times mild depression is well treated with good

nutrition, relaxation, and enhanced community or social support. But people on that treadmill of stress have little time and energy to invest in themselves or their families. Depression may worsen, taking a significant toll physically, mentally, and emotionally as well as leading to a reduction in productivity. Lack of treatment for depression leads to a bona fide health crisis.

Nutritional depletion

The third major factor for quality of life is nutrition because without it, disease is sure to follow. Clearly the American public is very interested in learning more about nutrition. Many bestsellers over the years have focused on nutrition and health. Pritikin, Atkins, the Zone Diet, Eat Right for Your Blood Type, and the South Beach Diet are household names for most Americans. But while some form of nutritional education has been available in mainstream medicine for years, nutrition has not been considered a cornerstone of a typical patient's therapy.

Setting aside the junk food epidemic, it is widely believed that foods eaten today are grown in soils that are depleted of nutrients. Even when we consume what appear to be healthy diets, we are not getting the FDA–recommended doses of vitamins and minerals in our food. Donald Davis, research associate with the Biochemical Institute at the University of Texas, Austin, analyzed data from the USDA in 1950 and 1999 on the nutritional content of forty-three fruit and vegetable crops. He learned that six of thirteen nutrients had noticeably declined in these crops over a fifty-year period.[74]

The decline in our produce's nutritional value corresponds to the period of increasing industrialization of our farming systems. As we have substituted chemical fertilizers, [and] pesticides...for the natural cycle of nutrients and on-farm biodiversity, we have lessened the nutritional value of our produce."[75]

The irony of this apparent nutritional depletion is the state of abundance of the U.S. food supply. "Americans enjoy one of the most plentiful and affordable food supplies in the world. With this abundance has come overconsumption—of calories, fat, sodium—and a host of related health conditions."[76]

"Human beings are genetically adapted to conditions of scarcity and irregular nutrition. In case of food abundance, this advantage turned into a significant part of the population's predisposition to 'diseases of civilization.'"[77] This conclusion was made by I. S. Liberman, doctor of sciences, quoted by Alpha Galileo, a leading online resource for European research in science, medicine, and technology.

Atherosclerosis, type II diabetes, primary hypertension, and obesity are known as diseases of civilization. In other words, throughout history mankind has been able to adapt to periods of lack of food intake. Our ancestors did not enjoy an abundance of food, but they had the ability to store food, including fats, and use food when needed. We, instead, do not burn up the food we store; instead, fats get deposited in our blood vessels, and we develop heart conditions and other diseases and become diabetic.

One of those diseases is obesity, and obesity rates are increasing in our children. Children with a body mass index (BMI) equal to or greater than the 95th percentile for gender and age are considered overweight. The number of children who meet these criteria is growing each year in the United States.

Childhood obesity has become a pandemic of our time.

An almost fourfold increase in childhood obesity in the past three decades, twice the asthma rates since the 1980s, and a jump in the number of attention deficit disorder cases are driving the growth of chronic illnesses according to researchers at Harvard University."[78]

James Perrin, professor of pediatrics at Harvard Medical School, warns, "We will see much greater expenditures for people in their 20s than we ever saw before, and no one is thinking how we should prepare for that."[79] As these chronic illnesses increase in younger and younger patients, the cost to society will rise as well.

Many doctors believe the rise in childhood obesity is a direct result of heavy consumption of fast food.

Genes may play a role...but environmental and social changes are behind the surge, researchers say. Modern life has brought more fast food, increased time spent indoors watching TV or playing on the computer, and dwindling community and family support."[80]

Children aren't the only ones battling obesity. Americans, it seems, are constantly trying to lose weight. The risks of obesity are both mental and physical in nature. Besides low self-esteem and social insecurity, physical problems abound, including high blood pressure, elevated cholesterol and triglycerides, increased risk of diabetes, heart disease, health complications, and shorter life spans. The CDC National Center for Health Statistics estimates 66.3 percent of Americans age twenty and over are overweight.[81]

Joseph Mercola, DO, board certified in family medicine and the author of the number-one ranked natural-health Web site in the world, quotes researchers in the University Hospital Hambur-Eppendorf, Germany, who found "so-called 'healthy' fast food alternatives to have the same effect on the cardiovascular system as standard fast food menus."[82] The study included intake of vegetarian burgers, lemon-flavored carbonated drink, salad, fruit, yogurt, and orange juice.

Dr. Mercola elaborates:

Fast-food restaurants are not in the business of serving organic, wholesome, nutrition-dense foods at dirt-cheap prices. But that's what you need if you're aiming for optimal health. You may not necessarily get it dirt cheap, but you can eat healthy even if you're on a budget. And after you figure in what you'll spend on health care once your health has been neglected, eating organic suddenly seems like the least expensive option.[83]

Eating organic provides an important solution for Americans. Charles Benbrook, chief scientist at the Organic Center and former executive director of the Board of Agriculture of the National Academy of Sciences, reviewed antioxidant levels in conventional and organic foods. He found "in 85%... [of] produce from organic farms had higher levels of antioxidants than did produce from conventional farms."[84] Antioxidants help protect the body from toxins that have been linked to degenerative diseases. Benbrook adds, "As someone that has been involved with science and science policy my whole life...I think the scientific case has been made for organic produce."[85]

But "organic foods don't do the whole trick.... Even organic foods are often picked before they have fully ripened, which affects nutritional quality."[86]

How many years of quality of life and billions of dollars will be saved every year by large-scale implementation of healthy nutrition in our current healthcare delivery system?

Aging

An obvious reason for increasing rates of chronic illness is the fact that we are an aging population. "Improvements in nutrition, public sanitation and hygiene, personal habits, biomedical technology and health services delivery have caused mortality declines throughout the world" and certainly in the United States.[87] Over the next thirty years, the number of Americans over the age of sixty-five and the population of those individuals older than eighty-five is expected to double.[88]

Most senior citizens have one or more chronic health challenge. And with our current health system geared to the treatment of acute health conditions, what do those seniors who have more than one chronic health challenge do?

Population aging, accelerating as the baby boom generations age, will have important fiscal consequences because expenditures on Social Security, Medicare and institutional Medicaid make up more than a third of the Federal budget" say Lee and Edwards in a paper written for the Center for the Economics and Demography of Aging, U.C., Berkeley.[89]

In "Healthy Aging v. Chronic Illness: Preparing Medicare for the New Health Care Challenges," David Kendall, et al., report "over three-quarters of the Medicare population suffers from one or more chronic conditions. In less than 20 years, care for these conditions will consume 80 percent of the nation's health care spending."[90]

Curtailing skyrocketing health costs of an aging population must address at least three areas.

1. A shift in healthcare services from acute- to chronic-care management.

As a conventional healthcare clinician, what I need most to offer my current patients are strategies to help them manage their chronic health conditions more effectively. Medications are simply not enough to help people with chronic health conditions live well and thrive.

Global Action on Aging, a nonprofit advocacy group for the elderly, based in New York at the United Nations, summarizes the chronic health challenges well:

> While modern medicine and public health have dramatically improved our ability to survive acute threats like heart attacks and infectious diseases, chronic conditions demand new and fundamentally different approaches...for well over a century, medicine has emphasized acute care. Doctors are trained to "find it and fix it." A broken bone needs a cast. A heart attack leads to a bypass operation to correct a clogged artery. A badly infected foot is amputated.... While obviously necessary in many cases, these medical responses often represent a failure to act *proactively* against chronic diseases, which are, by definition, ongoing and resistant to quick fixes.

> The failure to pay for better chronic care reflects a larger failure to pay for quality improvement in health care. Medicare's Industrial Age regulatory machinery inhibits its ability to innovate and adapt.... Entrenched attitudes, including the belief that poor health is an inevitable consequence of old age, further impede progress.[91]

Our conventional healthcare system limits what we offer patients to medications, more medications, and various medication combinations. Our patients with chronic health conditions suffer from pain, difficulty walking, weight problems, cravings for sweets and fast foods, sleep problems, anxiety, lightheadedness, fatigue, panic attacks, insecurity, fear, and low self-esteem. Yes, medications have their place but these patients need so much more.

According to Mokdad, et al., in the *Journal of the American Medical Association*:

Even though the statistics related to chronic illness are daunting, the U.S. health care system has been slow to espouse a system of care focused more on helping patients prevent and maintain chronic conditions, in order to improve outcomes and reduce costs. The aging of the population, combined with the growing epidemic of obesity and its fearsome cascade of increased diabetes, hypertension, and cardiovascular morbidity and mortality, demands the redesign of our health system to better help patients manage the chronic illnesses.[92]

The transformation of U.S. healthcare *must* thoroughly integrate prevention and early interventional strategies that address chronic health challenges; these approaches *must* occur swiftly for the sake of quality of life of older Americans and to prevent healthcare spending that our federal budget will not sustain in the long term.

2. Address the needs of an aging population for long-term care.

According to Mark McClellan, MD, PhD, administrator for the Centers for Medicare and Medicaid Services, "Our challenge today is to make sure long term care services are flexible and able to meet the different needs of a modern health care system."[93]

Dorcas Hardy, policy chairman of the White House Conference on Aging, describes a "coming of age" that "amplifies the urgent need of a balanced, integrated national long term care policy to meet the demands of a diverse older population that largely desires quality, individual choice, access and affordability."[94]

Nearly half of all Americans will need long-term care at some point in their lives. One in five over age fifty is at risk of needing it in the next twelve months.[95]

Two visits a day by a home health aide to help with bathing, dressing, and household chores can cost $2,500 a month, or more if skilled help such as physical therapy is needed.[96]

In the words of Karen Ignagni, president and CEO of American's Health Insurance Plans and ranked by *Modern Healthcare* magazine as among the one hundred most powerful people in healthcare:

> Our nation needs to broaden the healthcare discussion that has been focused on acute care to one that focuses on continuity of care that people need throughout their lives.... There needs to be a paradigm shift in the financing and delivery of health care that reflects twenty-first century realities of chronic illness and our aging population."[97]

Healthcare for an aging population must be proactive and affordable. Nursing and assisted living care is beyond the means of many hardworking Americans. It is essential that intense efforts be focused on keeping us healthy as a nation and finding ways to make longer term care affordable before it is too late.

3. The need to study and establish preventative measures for accidents and injury in an aging population.

Stewart C. Wang, MD, PhD, points to an increase in admissions by elderly patients in the University of Michigan Trauma Center.

> This trend toward more and more elderly trauma has been noted at other trauma centers and is likely to accelerate in the upcoming decades as the general population ages...currently 12.5% of the U.S. population over age 65 accounts for almost one-third of all deaths from injury and incurs a higher population based death rate than any other age group.[98]

Although the elderly drive less overall, the rate of motor vehicle crashes among that group is quite high, and according to Wang, "motor vehicle crashes are the most common reason for the elderly to be transported to a trauma center."[99]

Severity of bone fractures, diminished lung function and capacity, and an overall diminished ability of older individuals to heal make this rising health challenge a formidable issue in the aging U.S. population. Further studies are necessary to identify solutions that are preventative in nature, to prevent accidents and trauma, to enhance quality of life, and to curb skyrocketing healthcare costs.

Disabled Americans

Besides aging, rates of disabilities are rising in America. Recent data suggests that "as many as 50 million Americans currently live with physical or mental impairments that prevent them from taking on regular work or life activities."[100]

In "Report: U.S. Unready for Rise in Disabled," Todd Zwillich quotes Alan M. Jette, director of the Health and Disability Research Institute at Boston University, who warns, "It becomes quite clear that disability will essentially affect the lives of most Americans." Zwillich adds, "The report scolds U.S. policy makers for largely ignoring the coming consequences of disability." He quotes Jette: "The public could become galvanized by the large number of U.S. military personnel returning from wars in Iraq and Afghanistan with 'terrible disabilities.'"[101]

A recent study by the Physicians for Social Responsibility revealed "health care for veterans returning from the Iraq war could cost the U.S. as much as $650 billion, eventually exceeding the cost of combat operations."[102]

Many disabled Americans are strongly committed to enhanced health, wellness, and productivity in their lives. Our current "illness-based" healthcare system does not even begin to address these vital needs. A transformational healthcare system proactively promotes health and wellness in our disabled citizens, first to improve the quality of their lives and promote productivity and optimal functioning.

Any discussion on the rise of chronic illness would not be complete without close attention to the environment, the risk of environmental toxins, and the need for a long-term U.S. strategy to make environmental health and safety a top priority. These issues, of utmost importance, are addressed in the next chapter.

CHAPTER 5

Health, Illness, and the Environment

WE LIVE IN TIMES WHEN WE CAN NO LONGER afford to ignore the relationship between our environment and our health. The World Health Organization estimates that 23 percent of all deaths globally and 36 percent of deaths in children under age fourteen "are due to modifiable environmental factors."[103]

As far as health is concerned,

Many studies in people have demonstrated an association between environmental exposure and certain diseases...examples include radon and lung cancer; arsenic and cancer in several organs; lead and nervous system disorders; disease-causing bacteria such as E coli O57:H7 (e.g. contaminated meat and water) and gastrointestinal illness and death; and particulate matter and aggravation of heart and respiratory diseases.[104]

According to Philip R. Lee, MD, chairman of the Collaboration on Health and the Environment and former U.S. assistant secretary of Health and Human Services:

Compelling scientific evidence increasingly indicates that the proliferation of chemicals in our air, water, soil, food, homes, schools, and workplaces can be an important issue in many human diseases and health conditions.

The effects of such environmental toxicants can range from minor to severe. Increasing numbers of informed individuals and organizations are concerned about these impacts and attempting to learn more about the risks and options for minimizing or eliminating such exposures.

Unfortunately, such efforts in environmental health have too often been fragmented. Medical, patient, public health and environmental groups that share some of the same concerns often have not worked together towards common goals. A diverse and inclusive collaboration is essential in reducing public exposure to environmental toxicants and developing preventative strategies. Everyone concerned— health-affected groups, scientists, health professionals, and environmental organizations—can serve as resources for each other in collaborations that will help reduce public exposure to environmental toxicants.[105]

The Collaboration on Health and the Environment, a nonpartisan partnership, exists to "address growing concerns about the links between human health and the environment."[106] One resource available to the public is the CHE Toxicant and Disease Database, which includes 180 human diseases and ranks the risks of developing each disease to exposure to particular toxicants.

Sherry A. Rogers, MD, a diplomat of both the American Board of Family Practice and the American Board of Environmental Medicine, has spent years educating doctors and the public on these vital environmental issues.

The plastics encasing our foods—including those that contain almost all of the beverages we consume—and the Styrofoam cups we drink out of are two regular sources of environmental toxins. Rogers reminds us, "Studies show that plastic leaches right out of plastic wrap and into the foods where it stays until you ingest it."[107]

Rogers alerts us that plastics contain phthalates (plasticizers), which resemble hormones and mimic the effect of hormones in the body. They can cause symptoms of hor-

monal imbalance, including depression, mood swings, memory loss, and fatigue, as well as infertility and endometriosis. In addition, they can cause hormone-related cancers, including breast, testicular, and prostate cancer.[108]
Rogers reminds us:

> No one is saying that (the causes of all these diseases, including cancer) totally is due to plastics.... Plastics are just one minuscule example of the hundreds of environmental chemicals that we stockpile and that cause our diseases.... In addition to plastics, the EPA also found dioxins and PCBs in 100% of human fat samples. These two man-made chemicals are among the top most potent causes of cancer known to man. No wonder cancer has reached an all-time high as we all continually stockpile what we are unable to metabolize.[109]

Toxins are everywhere—in our carpets, in car fumes, in paint, in metals, in the air. The list is endless. The pesticides sprayed on our foods to *kill* pests are toxic to us as well. In the words of Bette Hileman, senior editor of *Chemical Engineering News*, "Over the past few decades disturbing trends have led researchers to believe that environmental exposures are contributing to children's declining health status in the U.S."[110]

According to a position paper by the National Environmental Health Association on Children's Environmental Health, "Children's systems are still developing.... They are more susceptible to environmental threats. Exposure to toxic substances can affect the growth of fetuses, infants and children.... Such exposures may impair development of children's nervous systems and cause abnormal development because of hormonal or immunologic effects."[111]

This position paper points to some startling statistics:

- Ten million children under the age of twelve live within 4 miles of a hazardous waste dump
- About half of all pesticides a person ingests in a lifetime are taken in by the age of five
- Asthma deaths increased in young people by 118 percent between 1980 and 1993; more than 25 percent of children in the United States live in areas that fail to meet national quality air standards[112]

Former U.S. Public Health Service Director Philip R. Lee says, "Environmental exposure to any a number of known and suspected developmental neurotoxins could contribute to ADHD, including lead, mercury, manganese, tobacco, smoke, polychlorinated biphenyls (PCBs), certain pesticides and solvents."[113]

According to Lee, "The impact of neurodevelopmental disorders such as ADHD on children is immense. Children with ADHD are at greater risk for dropping out of school early, drug abuse and suicide."[114]

Another childhood disorder correlated to exposure to environmental toxins—at least in part—is autism. Childhood autism is a disabling condition with onset typically before three or four years of age, occurring in an alarming 1 in every 150 children. Although controversy remains about the relationship between autism and environmental toxins, Martha Herbert, MD, PhD, assistant professor of neurology at Harvard Medical School and pediatric neurologist at Massachusetts General, says, "Observations about environmental factors relevant to autism go back decades."[115]

Herbert explains,

Currently chemicals are studied only one at a time.... A very large number of chemicals, those that were on the market before the institution of present regulations, have been 'grandfathered in,' that is, allowed to be marketed without testing.... Amazingly there is no requirement to test chemicals for their impacts on the developing nervous system, so that out of the approximately 3,000 chemicals produced in the largest volumes, *only 20–30* have been tested.... For the rest, the painful truth is that we are flying blind.[116]

According to a report from *Pediatrics* in 2006, comparing health utilization and costs of children with or without autism, researchers found substantially higher cost for children with autism. Average costs for hospitalizations, clinic visits, and prescription medication were more than double compared to children without autism.[117]

Michael Ganz, MS, PhD, Harvard School of Public Health, estimates that each individual with autism accrues $3.2 million in lifetime costs to society. Although childhood expenses are largely related to medical care, costs in adulthood are attributable to lost productivity and other indirect expenses.[118]

"The financial burden that this will place on our society is going to be just stunning, and that is really the wake-up call here," states Andy Shih, director of research and programs at the National Alliance for Autism Research.[119]

Another source of poisoning is lead. A recent report by MSNBC.com reveals that 35 percent of children's toys contain lead.[120] Children's toys were tested for lead, cadmium, and arsenic, among other toxic chemicals. Although many toys were recalled, how many toys in the hands of our children have *not* been tested and what is the health risk to our children?

Economics plays a large role in environmental issues. What is the balance between economic development and environmental safety? The issue of economics and the environment is complex and parallels the earlier issues regarding health and the role of technological innovation.

According to the Environmental Protection Agency, "Sustainable development marries two important themes: that environmental protection does not preclude economic development and that economic development must be ecologically viable now and in the future."[121]

The term "sustainability" gained popularity after the Brundtland Report defined sustainable development as "development that meets the needs of the present without compromising the ability of future generations to meet their own needs."[122]

A vital question is, why the issue of sustainability?

A poignant answer is found in the textbook *Sustainability and Health: Supporting Global Ecological Integrity in Public Health*: "When in 20 years' time one of my grandchildren asks me why our generation let things go on for so long when everything was telling them time was running out, I want to be able to tell them I did all I could."[123]

Environmental Defense is an American organization committed to a sustainable environment. Its mission is "dedicated to protecting the environmental rights of all people, including future generations. Among these rights are access to clean air and water, healthy and nourishing food, and flourishing ecosystems."[124]

A nonprofit organization with more than five hundred thousand members, Environmental Defense has, since 1967, "linked science, economics and law to create innovative, equitable and cost-effective solutions to society's most urgent environmental problems."[125]

Environmental health risks are targeted by Environmental Defense. One article warns of "increased hospital visits, disease and even death...associated with unusually high temperatures...and outbreaks of tropical diseases are expected to increase."[126]

In "Cleaning Up Dirty School Buses," Environmental Defense describes the health risks of the diesel engines that pollute the air inside the bus.

Diesel engines spew out nearly 40 toxic substances...coarse and fine particles are breathed deeply into the lungs where they can lodge, creating serious, even life-threatening problems...[such] as aggravated asthma, lung inflammation, heart problems, possible cancer, premature death."[127]

Likewise, Environmental Defense articulates the risks of toxic pollution from cars and trucks: "Asthma is the nation's fastest-growing chronic disease, afflicting more than 22 million Americans. Asthma rates among children more than doubled over the last twenty years."[128] "Some studies have found associations between traffic-related exposures and stroke, cancers, including childhood leukemias, and adverse reproductive outcomes."[129]

These facts clearly articulate the dire impact of ignoring environmental concerns on the health of Americans. It will take forethought, strategic planning, and concerted action to integrate many widely divergent fields that affect the environment and health.

Economically, corporations and stockholders are demanding sustainability information for their decision making, from purchasing products and services to making investments. Leaders in health transformation must make the same keen investment in the health of the American people and include environmentally sound strategies for any health initiatives to be effective. Let us be able to tell our children and grandchildren, "We did all we could *and* we made the world a much better place for you!"

As I discuss in the next chapter, Hippocrates supported the notion that nature—which includes the human body—could cure itself, and that the quality of the environment had an important bearing on this process. Hippocrates advocated environmental quality as a factor in keeping people healthy. Let's further examine why any health transformation initiatives must incorporate Hippocratic principles.

CHAPTER 6

The Hippocratic Oath

ALL MODERN PHYSICIANS TAKE THE Hippocratic Oath, which in essence tells them that in caring for patients, "do no harm."

According to Lee, Kliger, and Shiflett in "Integrative Medicine, Principles for Practice":

During the time that the Hippocratic Oath was written, around 300 BC, the philosophy of medicine reflected an emphasis on observation of all aspects of the individual, from diet to the nature and content of dreams, as a means of understanding the malady suffered by that individual. Hippocratic physicians were strongly encouraged to resist classifying diseases solely according to the organs affected. Each patient was seen as an individual rather than a "disease entity." The notion of an individual as a combination of both material and spiritual properties was an accepted medical paradigm.... A constant thread throughout the writings of this time was a reliance on nature, and the main objective of treatment was to help patients achieve harmony so that the natural forces in the body (humors) could return to a state of balance. Relief of suffering was primarily achieved by alterations in lifestyle, in diet, and the life of the spirit... The mind and the body were seen as inseparable parts contained within each person, each person a combination of physical and spiritual properties.[130]

How are practitioners embodying the Hippocratic Oath today? How is the conventional healthcare system promoting a doctor's ability to "do no harm" and to live up to the Hippocratic Oath?

Today, conventional medicine is the third leading cause of death in this country, after heart disease and cancer.[131] In an article in the *Journal of the American Medical Association*, Barbara Starfield, MD, summarizes several research studies in the last decade:

- 7,000 deaths per year from medication errors in hospitals
- 20,000 deaths per year from other errors in hospitals
- 80,000 deaths per year from infections in hospitals
- 106,000 deaths per year from negative effects from drugs

Practitioners in conventional healthcare have seen an exponential flurry of increased healthcare regulations in response to those horrifying statistics. We have already identified the costs of these increased healthcare regulations. Ironically, increased regulations on their own do not necessarily improve patient care or quality patient outcomes. Increased regulations translate into a steadily increasing stream of paperwork thrust on an already overburdened hospital or clinic staff. More paperwork means staff have less time to spend with patients.

We have also identified the almost complete lack of prevention and early intervention for patients with chronic health challenges in our current healthcare system. Yes, the United States is known as having the best acute and trauma care in the world. Ask any patient or family member of an accident victim to describe the miracles of modern medicine. If a car wreck occurs, an individual is skillfully removed from the automobile and transferred via helicopter, if necessary, to a level I trauma facility. This individual may leave like a new person, thanks largely to the incredible skill of surgeons, intensive care units, and their highly dedicated staff. We cannot minimize the role of the emergency response teams and their heroic efforts and skill.

These are the miracles of modern medicine today. And yes, they do happen.

Every day.

The flaws in our current system are probably best measured, not by what is being done, but on what is virtually absent. For the last century, there has been a near absence of Hippocratic principles, except those in regard to patient confidentiality.

There is little meaningful education on nutrition, although Hippocrates so astutely stated, "Let your food be your medicine, and your medicine be your food." The speed in our current healthcare system has all but replaced a meaningful solution focused on a health-sustaining relationship between patient and healthcare practitioner.

Our conventional healthcare setting limits disease recovery to processes controlled by medications and surgeries. It focuses on one aspect of healing—destroying the disease. While fighting off disease with medications and surgeries, our cells quickly become exhausted.

Sickness is like a war going on in our bodies. Medications fight illness with pinpoint precision. But fighting illness is an exhausting job. The ill effects of warding off illness linger long after the illness is gone; cells are depleted from within and lack the resources to remain healthy.

Cells, after fighting illness, are like batteries running on their last bits of power. The body is at risk of giving out and experiencing a meltdown of its natural defense mechanisms. Think about why so many people today complain of feeling exhausted—their immune systems have never fully recovered.

Rather than treat the whole person, as Hippocrates advocated, our conventional system is driven by procedures that lead to diagnosis and treatments without regard for the long-term processes involved in healing. Insurance companies reimburse for a five- to ten-minute medication management visit. No codes exist for a health and wellness consultation that would integrate CAM therapies designed to promote long-term healing.

Millions of Americans are using CAM and experiencing its benefits—feeling better, reducing side effects of medications, decreasing hospitalizations, and lowering the numbers of medications needed daily. How do I know? For years I've been listening to people from all socioeconomic classes and walks of life. I can tell you what I see and what I know. If CAM didn't help, people would have stopped using it a long time ago. People want to feel well, be productive, and enjoy life. And what is unhealthy about that?

Likewise, I've talked to many conventional healthcare doctors who hear the same success stories from their patients. I hear them say they ethically can no longer sit passively while so many more patients could benefit from integrating CAM into their conventional healthcare. We took an oath.

Doctor-patient relationship

To practice Hippocratic principles, a doctor needs to listen carefully to the patient and see the patient as a whole person. This is in contrast to our current healthcare system, which is disease- and organ-specific with little regard to "the sum of the parts."

In "The Decline in the Patient-Physician Relationship," Quattrini writes:

> Over the span of half a century, the medical profession has witnessed a catastrophic shift in the patient-physician relationship. As...the number of patients under a doctor's care continues to rise, doctors are finding it hard to employ the time-honored principles listed within the Hippocratic Oath.... Hippocrates believed that it was the physician's duty, as a healer, to treat the patient infected with the disease to the best of his ability...the patient was, above all, the most important aspect involved in the healing process.[132]

Medical schools are beginning to require courses and training in doctor-patient communication and to establish physician requirements for graduation and licensure.[133]

Transforming the nature of the doctor-patient relationship is an essential element of *consumer-driven healthcare.* "Increased consumer control of health care is shaking up the medical and insurance systems."[134] Hospitals, doctors, benefits administrators, accountants, government policymakers, and insurers must adapt or they will be replaced.[135]

A fundamental premise of consumer-driven healthcare is listening to what consumers want from their healthcare system before meaningful reforms can take place.

Conclusion

Changes in healthcare must include restoration of Hippocratic principles in the daily practice of medicine.

CAM, as discussed in the next chapter, offers a wide array of options designed for prevention and early intervention for people with chronic disease. A competent integrative health doctor can offer many strategies to patients currently cared for by conventional medicine. These natural modalities are designed to boost the immune system, prevent relapse, and help reduce unwanted side effects from the conventional treatments.

And we cannot underestimate the value of good nutrition for healing and restoration. Good nutrition is a hallmark of good health and needed by the body to fight off infection, get well, and stay well. Extra nourishment is provided from high-quality nutritional supplements, either to prevent illness or help restore people to a state of health after protracted illness.

CHAPTER 7

Understanding Complementary and Alternative Medicine

I SEE PATIENTS EVERY DAY WHO ARE ASKING for more from their healthcare than medications. They are on medications and engaged in good therapy, but it is not enough. Daily, patients are asking for guidance on issues of low energy, burnout, insomnia, chronic pain, anxiety, restlessness, and stress management. These patients are asking for complementary and alternative medicine (CAM).

The second major healthcare system in the United States, CAM, is "a group of diverse medical and health systems, practices and products that are not presently considered to be a part of conventional medicine."[136] CAM consists of several components, which I discuss in this chapter.

A study released in May 2004 by the National Center for Complementary and Alternative Medicine revealed that 36 percent of U.S. adults eighteen or older use some form of CAM. When prayer is included in the definition of CAM, the number of adults using some form of CAM rose to 62 percent.[137]

Complementary medicine and alternative medicine are theoretically distinct and separate forms of treatment. Complementary medicine refers to treatments used in addition to conventional medical therapies, such as using medication along with massage therapy.

Alternative medicine refers to treatments that are used instead of conventional medicine, such as the systems of care like naturopathy, homeopathy, or ayurvedic medicine. With the advent of integrative medicine, however, even alternative medicine is being used more and more in conjunction with mainstream conventional medicine.

CAM is defined by the White House Commission on Complementary and Alternative Medicine Policy as

> a group of medical, health care, and healing systems other than those included in mainstream health care in the United States. CAM includes the worldviews, theories, modalities, products and practices associated with these systems and their use to treat illness and promote health and well-being.[138]

For our discussion, all CAM has the potential to be used in conjunction with conventional medicine when deemed safe and appropriate by a trained integrative health practitioner.

The National Center for Complementary and Alternative Medicine (NCCAM), founded in October 1998, is the federal government's lead agency for scientific research on CAM. NCCAM is one of twenty-seven institutes that make up the National Institutes of Health (NIH) within the U.S. Department of Health and Human Services. The U.S. government has been very supportive of CAM and CAM research, and of sharing this knowledge with health practitioners.

NCCAM's mission is to "explore complementary and alternative healing practices in the context of rigorous science, train complementary and alternative medicine researchers, and disseminate authoritative information to the public and professionals."[139]

NCCAM currently defines five major categories of CAM practices:

1. Whole medical systems, such as homeopathy, naturopathic medicine, ayurveda, and Chinese medicine
2. Mind-body medicine, including prayer and meditation
3. Biologically based practices including herbs and nutritional supplements

4. Manipulative and body-based practices including chiropractic and massage
5. Energy medicine, involving the use of energy fields (i.e., Reiki, therapeutic touch, use of electromagnetic fields)

Conventional medicine and CAM

Many doctors like myself have witnessed the benefits of integrating CAM into patients' day-to-day lives. Many have seen such considerable benefits that not speaking to the issues of incorporating CAM violates the Hippocratic Oath they took to become a physician. In other words, we as doctors can no longer remain silent when resources in CAM are available to help our patients and we have no access to these resources and we practice in a healthcare environment that does not even acknowledge CAM exists.

Today a conventional doctor needs to know about CAM. Many patients come to the office with excellent questions about CAM or having tried CAM therapies. Patients are eager to know which CAM therapies may work with their conventional health treatments. Many chronically ill patients describe being tired of trying numerous conventional treatments with no or partial success. Others have suffered significant side effects from their medications. It seems knowledge and access to CAM would greatly support a doctor's efforts in promoting health and caring for patients.

Today's physician needs to be well versed in integrating CAM in conventional practice. In "What Doctors Should Know about CAM," Alvarez and Murakumi write:

There are studies to show that CAM is beneficial for acute and chronic conditions as well as for preventative health care. When used to treat acute conditions, such as labor pain, postpartum depression, pregnancy-induced and chemotherapy-induced nausea, and surgical or procedural pain, CAM therapies work by affecting pain receptors, improving immune function, producing pharmacologic effects, increasing endorphin release, adjusting spine or manipulating muscle tissue.... Chronic conditions that have been reported to improve with the use of alternative therapies include cardiovascular disease, hypertension, asthma, ulcers, HIV and acquired immunodeficiency syndrome (AIDS), epilepsy, anxiety, depression, insomnia, back pain, headaches, and drug and alcohol addiction.[140]

If this information is available, why is CAM not approved for use in our conventional healthcare system? The chronic health conditions named that have been helped by CAM are serious conditions—AIDS, epilepsy, and cardiovascular disease to name a few. Can we not afford to research CAM further and incorporate CAM into our mainstream practices?

The Substance Abuse and Mental Health Services Administration (SAMHSA), a division of the U.S. Department of Health and Human Services, has included Alternative Approaches to Mental Health Care in its National Mental Health Information Center, which includes: self-help, diet and nutrition, pastoral counseling, animal-assisted therapies, expressive therapies (art, dance/movement, music/sound), culturally based healing arts (acupuncture, ayurveda, yoga, meditation, Native American traditional practices, cuentos), relaxation and stress-reduction techniques (biofeedback, massage therapy, guided imagery, visualization), and technology-based applications (telemedicine, telephone, counseling, electronic communications, radio psychiatry).[141]

According to the White House Commission on Complementary and Alternative Medicine Policy,

> Because of the dramatic increase in the prevalence of chronic conditions, the past decade has witnessed an acceleration both in consumer interest in and use of CAM practices and/or products. Surveys indicate that those with the most serious and debilitating medical conditions, such as cancer, chronic pain, and HIV, tend to be the most frequent users of CAM practices.[142]

I was surprised—and pleased—to learn that the White House Commission on Complementary and Alternative Medicine Policy even existed. After reading the commission's final report, I believe it provides the backbone for the development of an entirely transformed U.S. healthcare system.

Regardless of how a doctor may feel about CAM therapies, patients are using the treatments and finding success.

> Over the past 30 years, public interest in and use of complementary and alternative medicine (CAM)...has risen steadily in the United States. Depending on how CAM is defined...as much as 43% of the U.S. population has used some form of CAM.[143]

Why patients use CAM therapies

I've spoken to hundreds of patients over the years who tell me that medicines and surgeries are simply "not enough" to get well and stay well. These are the patients who explore and research all available avenues to improve the quality of their health. These are the patients who use CAM on a very regular basis.

In "Why Patients Use Alternative Medicine," John Astin states:

> Along with being more educated and reporting poorer health status, the majority of alternative medicine users appear to be doing so not so much as being dissatisfied with conventional medicine, but largely because they find these health care alternatives to be more congruent with their own values, beliefs and philosophical orientations toward health and life.[144]

According to the American Academy of Pediatrics, CAM is used frequently for children as well. For years I've worked with parents of children with special needs. I have never met a more proactive group of people dedicated to their children's health and well-being. Why are parents seeking CAM for their children? The parents I talk to are invariably not totally satisfied with conventional treatment. Even when it is working, it is simply not enough. Parents are looking for ways to integrate nutrition and wellness into the daily lives of their children. They are concerned about the short- and long-term side effects of medication. Many are already integrating CAM into their childrens' day-to-day lives.

Pediatric use of CAM is especially likely among children with chronic illness or disability. Up to 50% of children with autism in the United States are probably using some form of CAM...increasingly pediatricians providing care for children with chronic illness or disability are discussing CAM with families."[145]

Chronic illnesses in children for which CAM is used include cystic fibrosis, cancer, arthritis, asthma, autism, attention-deficit disorder (ADD), as well as respiratory problems, headaches, and nosebleeds.

Children diagnosed with attention-deficit disorder in the United States are being prescribed stimulants at increasing rates. However, doctors like Zoltan Rona, M.D.,[146] who served as past president of the Canadian Holistic Medical Association, offers parents natural solutions and preventative strategies for children with not only ADD and other behavior challenges, but with asthma, allergies, and ear infections.

A CAM approach is incorporated into the total care offered at ADD Health and Wellness Centers, Inc., which offers comprehensive assessment and treatment for youngsters with ADD. Treatments include nutritional counseling and supplementation; medication if indicated; and sixteen hours of selected therapies that may include coaching, therapy, couples/family counseling, social skills training, school meetings, and parent training.

Shouldn't such wellness approaches become our standard of care for our young people?

CAM and detoxification

CAM plays a vital role in helping the body cleanse itself of toxins that are ingested in foods, as well as those assimilated from environmental pollutants. Dr. Baker summarizes CAM's role in this process of detoxification:

One of the principle goals of complementary therapies is to rid the body of accumulated wastes and toxins. Detoxification and cleansing are central to the healing process. CAM practitioners believe that toxins block the flow of vital energy. Free flow of this energy throughout the body is integral to maintaining good health.[147]

I still hear colleagues who dismiss the concept of detoxification. The principle just makes good common sense, and in a world full of environmental pollutants and toxins, it is one we need to integrate into the mainstream practice of medicine today.

What is the role of CAM in a transformational health system?

Patients and doctors are experiencing the benefits of CAM when it is used in conjunction with conventional medicine. As we will soon see, a transformational health system includes integrating CAM into a mainstream healthcare system that, in addition to being accountable philosophically and ethically to patients and doctors, is accountable fiscally as well. If CAM can keep our people healthy and help restore health in people who are ill—and lower healthcare costs—then what are we waiting for?

CHAPTER 8

Transformational Health: Case Studies

TODAY, MILLIONS OF AMERICANS USE an integrative approach in dealing with chronic illness. Let's visit with three such individuals and witness integrative health in action. As in previous case studies, these individuals' names have been changed to preserve the confidentiality of their identities.

Ruth

Ruth is among 5 percent of the U.S. population diagnosed with asthma. At forty-five years of age, she has had two hospitalizations in her lifetime for an acute asthma attack, has had numerous ER visits, and has been on inhalers since childhood. Since her early twenties, she seemed to require the inhalers more and has, over the years, required oral steroids. Ruth's asthma is considered moderate type because her symptoms are exacerbated with talking, and she becomes easily agitated during an attack.

Ruth's father was killed in a construction-related accident around the time she was diagnosed with asthma. She had always been Daddy's little girl and has fond memories of sitting on his lap and going places with him. She readily admits she never got over losing her dad.

Ruth currently lives with her mother, and several brothers and their families live nearby. She was married once to a man who cheated on her, and she subsequently divorced him. She has no children. She has been a teacher since her late twenties, but because of her increasing asthma symptoms, Ruth limits her work to substitute teaching.

Ruth has several friends from the school where she worked full-time for ten years. They live nearby and keep in touch regularly. She occasionally volunteers for community projects for underprivileged children.

Ruth's friends have been concerned about Ruth's increasing use of oral steroid medication. They also are concerned about some unprovoked outbursts on Ruth's part, including tearfulness and depression. One of her friends, a massage therapist, advised Ruth to look into more natural therapies to offset the likely side effects of the oral steroids. Ruth is open to this and has started reading about such therapies. She recently joined an asthma support group where she has met numerous people with asthma who use complementary and alternative medicine.

Ruth is like millions of Americans who look to CAM as a result of concerns about side effects of their conventional medication.

According to Leonard Bielory, MD, director of the Asthma and Allergy Research Center at New Jersey Medical School, "Only 10% to 30% of our health care is actually delivered by what we consider conventional or biomedical-oriented practitioners."[148]

Through participation in her support group, Ruth realized she had never resolved her grief over losing her father. She joined an experiential grief group at her local hospital, where art, music, storytelling, and writing are used to help participants work through unresolved grief issues. Ruth was able to identify emotional triggers to asthma attacks and learn positive coping skills to redirect her thoughts and emotions before an asthma attack ensues.

Ruth also started looking at nutritional triggers to her asthma attacks. She admitted to snacking on comfort foods when home in the evening, including chocolate and nuts. She even admitted to being a "junk food–aholic," especially during the holidays, when she would eat large amounts of any sweets or starchy foods that were in the house. Ruth decided to combat her cravings for comfort foods by having lots of fresh fruits and vegetables to munch on in the evenings. Ruth also learned about a Finnish study that confirmed the benefits of weight-management programs for people with asthma. She and some members of her support group joined the Y and embarked on a gradual but beneficial exercise regimen. Starting slowly was absolutely necessary so as not to trigger an asthma attack. Finding an exercise regimen that did not induce an asthma attack was tricky, ultimately Ruth joined a yoga class. Again, she started slowly, but learned quickly that the breathing techniques really helped her feel better. She used the breathing techniques when at home and under stress, whenever a trigger came up.

Ruth heard about a counselor who specialized in grief and teaching relaxation and stress reduction strategies, so Ruth began seeing the counselor for therapy. The counseling was intense, but after a period of almost one year, she felt tremendously better and rarely relied on inhalers or oral medications to control her asthma attacks. Ruth continues on a maintenance exercise regimen, has lost 25 pounds in three years, and feels great. With her increased energy levels, she socializes more with her friends and volunteers regularly at a women's shelter as a lay counselor.

Sarah

Sarah is a twenty-eight-year-old student studying for a PhD. She has been accepted for a teaching position at the same university where she earned her degree. She was selected from hundreds of candidates across the country. When a close friend asked how she felt, her eyes welled up with tears as she whispered, "I just want to feel better."

Sarah was diagnosed with fibromyalgia in her early twenties. Although she always excelled in school, she was limited in her physical activity by her disorder. When she started experiencing pain, she went to her doctor, who ran extensive blood tests and ruled out many other conditions. She was told by her doctor that fibromyalgia was a disorder of exclusion with diagnosis made when the tests run for all other conditions were negative.

Sarah learned about the pressure points of pain that are a hallmark of fibromyalgia, and she experienced fifteen of eighteen possible painful points. Her pain persisted for months on end and was often accompanied by joint stiffness. Sarah was equally frustrated by her persistent fatigue, even though she slept eight hours per night. Her sleep was often interrupted, however, by bursts of restless legs, which were very uncomfortable.

Sarah noticed increased symptoms of temporo-mandibular joint disorder (TMJ), which included more pain and jaw joint stiffness when she experienced higher levels of stress. Headaches during those periods of stress were common as well.

Sarah had tried numerous medications, including antidepressants such as Prozac and Elavil, as well as muscle relaxants; she did not like the side effects and was unable to focus effectively on her academics. She sought help from complementary and alternative medicine to alleviate her symptoms and to learn better ways of reducing stress, which she knew greatly exacerbated her pain.

She began a workout regimen in her school gym, but given her intense nature, she quickly realized she had gone too far too fast by diving into a high-intensity aerobic workout, which just made her pain unbearable. She discussed her symptoms with one of the instructors, who described the relief his wife, also a sufferer of fibromyalgia, found though the use of tai chi and yoga. Sarah enrolled in a yoga class and experienced benefits within several months.

Stress reduction and relaxation techniques were also helpful for Sarah. Practicing the art of mindfulness—living in the moment—helped alleviate a lot of worries and pressures Sarah admits placing on herself. Coming from a hard-driving, professional family, she internalized many of the same expectations, yet struggled with a lack of self-confidence, believing subconsciously that no matter what she accomplished it was never enough.

Although Sarah was not overweight, her food intake consisted of convenience foods and snacks without regard for nutritional intake. Sarah reevaluated everything she ate and changed her eating habits dramatically for the better.

Today Sarah is teaching classes that she loves. She is almost completely pain-free and is off all medications. She is engaged, has good friends, works out, and lives a rewarding and fulfilling life.

Dan

Dan is a fifty-year-old retired U.S. Army soldier who works full-time for his brother's real estate company. Dan is on numerous medications for high blood pressure, high cholesterol, diabetes, and gout; in addition, he has been on and off narcotic pain medications for several war injuries. He has been on antidepressants for several years as well. He is at least 70 pounds overweight, and in his own words, "If I stopped eating tomorrow, it would take me years to lose all this weight!" Dan's injuries to his legs, knees, feet, and spine have curtailed his activity level.

Although his wife is very health conscious and prepares healthy dinners, Dan admits to splurging on greasy breakfasts and large lunch portions with plenty of chips and sweets. At night, against his wife's wishes, he indulges in several shots of vodka or rum and falls asleep early. Fortunately, he has never shown up intoxicated for work or driven under the influence of alcohol.

Dan's wife is a holistic health nurse who sets up wellness programs and runs groups at a local assisted-living facility. Although she is very supportive of helping Dan design a wellness program, she feels like her efforts had fallen on deaf ears—at least until Dan suffered his second heart attack.

Dan's doctor was kind but firm with him in the hospital. "You're going to have to bite the bullet and get this lifestyle thing under control, my friend." Dan knew exactly what his doctor was talking about. He felt like he was caught in a cycle of bad habits and was in a rut that he couldn't get himself out of. In the hospital, he had several good talks with his wife and implored her help. He knew he couldn't do this alone.

In addition, he joined Alcoholics Anonymous (AA). He got a sponsor to help ensure accountability twenty-four hours a day, seven days a week. He developed a new group of friends he could join for breakfast and had his wife help him pack healthy lunches. Often she would join Dan for a light lunch, and they would go for a walk afterward, weather permitting. With her encouragement, he met with a nutritionist and enrolled in a gym and got a personal trainer.

Dan had witnessed some tragic violent episodes in his neighborhood when he was a teenager. He had never resolved this and felt like he should have done more, and as result, has been very hard on himself. He started counseling with a therapist who helped him see that he had internalized a lifetime's worth of pain and was eating and drinking to numb himself. Gradually, with support and guidance, he learned to let go of his guilt, frustration, and low self-worth, and he started living in gratitude for all the wonderful things he has in his life.

Dan is doing well. He has lost 40 pounds in one year, his relationship with his wife is stronger than ever, and he hasn't needed any narcotic pain meds in almost twelve months. He has been able to gradually reduce the doses of his medications because of his improved physical status. He has had no gout flare-ups, and his primary-care doctor is giving him a thumbs-up for a job well done this past year for getting his health—and his life—back on track.

Conclusion

Each person discussed has very different health challenges, yet the solutions have much in common. Ruth, Sarah, and Dan each needed to examine the psychological factors affecting their health, and they all needed good nutritional support, a regular exercise regimen, and a strong social support network to help restore the quality of their lives and health.

CHAPTER 9

Educating Doctors for the Twenty-First Century

DOCTORS OF THE FUTURE—THOSE WHO ARE committed to the practice of the Hippocratic Oath—have had to be self-taught, proactive, and flexible in their approach to patient care. Because conventional doctors do not have established standards for the practice of integrative medicine, they have had to learn specifics regarding CAM and natural health from listening to their patients and from doctors with more experience than they.

Doctors of the future are learning about integrative medicine from the following sources:

- Institute for Functional Medicine
- Andrew Weil's Program for Integrative Medicine
- American Academy of Environmental Medicine
- National Center for Complementary and Alternative Medicine (a division of the National Institutes of Health)
- Center for Mind-Body Medicine

These organizations have much to offer in helping craft health-care solutions; let's not forget about them as healthcare is heatedly debated in the next few years.

The Institute for Functional Medicine

This nonprofit organization has a mission "to improve patient outcomes through prevention, early assessment, and comprehensive management of complex, chronic disease."[149]

What is functional medicine? Answers can be found on the home page of the Institute for Functional Medicine (www.functionalmedicine.org):

Functional medicine is personalized medicine that deals with primary prevention and underlying causes instead of symptoms for serious chronic disease. It is a science-based field of health care... **Functional medicine** is anchored by an examination of the core clinical imbalances that underlie various disease conditions. Those imbalances arise as **environmental inputs** such as diet, nutrients (including air and water), exercise, and trauma **are processed** by one's body, mind, and spirit through a unique set of genetic predispositions, attitudes, and beliefs.[150]

Our national research establishment—both private and governmental—is heavily focused on drug development and medical technology, rather than multifactorial, individualized, lifestyle-focused interventions. Even our less commercial research models all too often concentrate on single disease–single agent–single outcome methodologies.

This new understanding of the development of chronic diseases can and must be learned and implemented by U.S. physicians. The principles of functional medicine have not yet been adopted by most U.S. insurance companies. If they were, chances are high that health costs could be reduced by millions, possibly billions, of dollars.

It is imperative that world-class MDs and PhDs who contribute to the Institute for Functional Medicine's educational materials be consulted on U.S. health-care reform initiatives. It also seems essential that the quality preventative health-care training offered by the Institute for Functional Medicine become standards of care for licensed practicing physicians along with the more illness-based treatments.

The University of Arizona
Program in Integrative Medicine

The Fellowship in Integrative Medicine, founded and directed by Andrew Weil, is the primary education program at the University of Arizona Program in Integrative Medicine. The program's mission is "to lead the transformation of health care by creating, educating, and actively supporting a community of professionals who embody the philosophy and practice of integrative medicine."[151] Integrative medicine is defined as follows:

> Healing-oriented medicine that takes account of the whole person (body, mind, and spirit), including all aspects of lifestyle. It emphasizes the therapeutic relationship and makes use of all appropriate therapies, both conventional and alternative."[152]

The program consists of a comprehensive learning program for doctors, nurse practitioners, and physician assistants.

> Fellows of the Program learn to incorporate the philosophies and techniques of IM into their clinical practices, advance research in the field and create and lead academic programs, while becoming an agent of change in a worldwide community of integrative practitioners.[153]

The training is intense but worthwhile for the health-care practitioner who attends and for the patients cared for afterward. In fact, the demand for such doctors and health practitioners is very high, underscoring the needs and wishes of patients, particularly those with chronic health challenges.

Weil has pioneered an integrative medicine approach for years, and it is time these practices were integrated into a meaningful health-reform strategy for the United States.

American Academy of Environmental Medicine

The American Academy of Environmental Medicine (AAEM) is a nonprofit organization committed to "providing tools to recognize, evaluate, treat and prevent those aspects of illness caused by the role of the environment and diet."[154]

AAEM trains physicians through in-depth education and continuing medical education courses.

The doctors and health care practitioners that practice environmental medicine provide a comprehensive, patient-centered, preventative approach to medical care dedicated to the evaluation, management, and prevention of the adverse consequences of environmentally triggered illnesses.[155]

Up until recently, environmental medicine was not taught in medical schools and in fact was not widely accepted by conventional medicine. Though the efforts of AAEM, however, this is changing, and the field of environmental medicine emerging.

AAEM-trained physicians need to be included in U.S. health-reform initiatives.

National Center for Complementary and Alternative Medicine

The National Center for Complementary and Alternative Medicine (NCCAM) is the federal government's lead agency for scientific research on complementary and alternative medicine. NCCAM is one of twenty-seven institutes and centers that make up the National Institutes of Health (NIH) within the U.S. Department of Health and Human Services. As stated in Public Law 105-277, NCCAM's purpose is "the conduct and support of basic and applied research...research training, the dissemination of health information, and other programs with respect to identifying, investigating, and validating complementary and alternative treatment, diagnostic and prevention modalities, disciplines and systems."[156]

The organization's mission is as follows:
- Explore complementary and alternative healing practices in the context of rigorous science
- Train complementary and alternative medicine researchers
- Disseminate authoritative information to the public and professionals

NCCAM provides a wealth of scientific information for doctors who want to learn more about complementary and alternative medicine. Congress established the Office of Alternative Medicine in 1992 and the National Centers for Complementary and Alternative Medicine in 1999. NCCAM's 2007 budget was 121.4 million dollars, up from a 1999 budget of 50 million dollars.

NCCAM has four primary areas of focus:
1. *Advancing scientific research:* NCCAM has funded more than 1,200 research projects in the United States and worldwide.
2. *Training CAM researchers:* NCCAM supports training for new researchers and encourages experienced researchers to study CAM.
3. *Sharing news and information:* CAM research is disseminated though its continuing medical education courses, Web site, and publications.
4. *Supporting integration of proven CAM therapies:* CAM research helps the public and health professionals understand which CAM therapies have been proven to be safe and effective.

Approved research projects are diverse and cover CAM's integration in treating diseases such as multiple sclerosis, arthritis, coronary heart disease, and diabetes, among others.

A recent stakeholder's dialogue held at the NIH campus in Bethesda, Maryland, resulted in numerous suggestions for research.

Because CAM and integrative medicine are widely used by many Americans, research to determine the effectiveness and safety of promising treatment should be given high priority. NCCAM should fund more research on health promotion, disease prevention, wellness and integrative health care.[157]

According to one participant, "Don't focus on what's wrong with us and how to fix it...but on what's right with us and how to keep enhancing it.... We are interested in optimal health not just survival."[158]

Shouldn't members of NCCAM, an agency established by Congress and commissioned with educating people about CAM therapies, be invited by Congress to help craft health-policy reform?

Center for Mind-Body Medicine

Founded in 1991 by James S. Gordon, MD, the Center for Mind-Body Medicine (CMBM) is a nonprofit organization "dedicated to reviving the spirit and transforming the practice of medicine. The Center is working to create a more effective, comprehensive, and compassionate model of health-care and health education. The center's model combines the precision of modern science with the wisdom of the world's healing traditions, to help health professionals heal themselves, their patients and clients, and their communities."[159]

CMBM offers comprehensive training for doctors and allied health professionals. Included are continuing education courses on food as medicine, which integrates nutrition into clinical practice and medical education and Cancer Guide, the first comprehensive training in integrative oncology. The course teaches health professionals and patient advocates how to make the best choices in complementary and alternative medicine, as well as conventional forms of cancer treatment.

CMBM offers global outreach programs, including programs in Israel and Palestine, to train local leaders to offer mind-body medicine techniques to citizens suffering from trauma and stress from living in war conditions. Similar programs are being planned in the Gaza Strip, Kosovo, and New Orleans.

Dr. Gordon also served as the chairman of the White House Commission on Complementary and Alternative Medicine policy. According to the Center's founder,

> Over the last 30 years, increasing numbers of Americans, particularly those with chronic and life-threatening illnesses, have begun to look for health

care approaches in complementary and alternative approaches. They are not turning their back on conventional medicine—it is, in fact, those who have had all the benefits of modern scientific medicine who have led the search—but they are very much aware of its limitations and side effects. They are exploring approaches that would complement this medicine-or in some cases, be alternatives to it. And most often, they are exploring these approaches without valid scientific information to guide them.[160]

Credible sources of physician training on integrating complementary and alternative medicine into mainstream practice do exist. It is time these organizations play a role in crafting health transformation policy for all Americans.

CHAPTER 10

And Back to the Political Debates

I HOPE IT IS BECOMING MORE CLEAR that the current political debate over healthcare is largely a debate over *who* will administer the healthcare of the American public rather than how to maintain the good health of the American people. The current healthcare debates do not address the principles of healthcare related to wellness, preventing illness, and supporting cellular health for people *after* they become ill. Nor do the debates target the current healthcare administrative excesses (billions of dollars per year) and the profit motives that drive the research and development of pharmaceuticals and technology.

But be that as it may, let's review the salient points largely driving the current health reform dialogue:

Private healthcare vs. single-payer healthcare

Let's examine the pros and cons of private and single-payer healthcare models. In addition, let us examine questions of critical importance that have not met the national agenda—but must!

Private Healthcare Model = Private Insurance Healthcare

PROS:
Based on free markets

Allows for patient access to latest technology

Based on doctor/consumer freedom of choice

Allows the option of universal healthcare with freedom of choice

CONS:
Third-party managed care often restricts or denies benefits

High deductibles and co-pays

Many small businesses cannot afford

Minimal access to wellness services

Minimal access to nutritional supplements

Too costly for many Americans

Minimal input from citizens or doctors

Single-Payer Healthcare = Government-Sponsored Healthcare

PROS:
All people will be insured

The federal government will underwrite health insurance for all Americans

CONS:
Care will be likely be "cheaper" (i.e., primarily generic medication, less access to advanced health technology)

Taxes will likely be considerably higher

Administrative costs as great and probably higher

May still have same third-party managed care restricting and denying benefits

Rationing and denial of care Minimal access to wellness services

Minimal access to nutritional supplements

Questionable monies for health research

Most citizens agree that the current model of U.S. healthcare is failing. But what about the risks of single-payer healthcare? Goodman, Musgrave, and Herrick examined single-payer national health insurance around the world. Some of what they learned was very surprising:

1. "Even Canada has changed, using the United States as a partial safety valve for its overtaxed health care system; provincial governments and patients spend more than $1 billion on U.S. medical care."[161]
2. "We know of no country in the world that has established a universal right to any particular health care service. The one exception is the United States....[162] Citizens of Canada, for example, have no right to any particular health care service. They have no right to an MRI scan....They do not even have the right to a place in line."[163]
3. "The Canadian press is replete with the names of victims of rationing or inadequate care."[164] "In most countries with waiting lists for care, the poor wait longer than the wealthy and powerful."[165]
4. "...The proportion of Canadians satisfied with their health care system dropped from 56 percent to 20 percent between 1987 and 1997...it appears that people almost everywhere feel their health care system needs to be reformed...."[166]

I have personally talked to numerous Canadian citizens who reiterate the above concerns. In addition, many Canadians are eager to integrate prevention and wellness into their healthcare system but tend to believe this will happen here in the United States faster than in Canada.

It appears that all healthcare systems are stressed and in need of reform. Rather than change the U.S. health delivery system from private to single payer at this time, it seems far more prudent and cost-effective to invest in prevention and wellness *first* rather than reform an already broken system. I hope the risks of a sudden switch to single-payer healthcare are evident. How can we add billions of dollars of additional health expenditures before we drastically reduce current excess healthcare costs and expenditures?

"Single payer" refers to government-sponsored healthcare, with premiums derived primarily from tax dollars. Without curtailing healthcare expenditures, the rates of tax increases for the average American will be staggering in the next three to ten years. Add that to an already stressed economy, with citizens struggling to balance mortgage payments, food, and gas bills, it seems most sensible to lower health expenditures and actively study and implement health, wellness, and prevention to reduce the need for people to need higher priced medical care after they become ill. Then and only then will it be the time to make a collective decision as to the model of healthcare we desire as Americans.

So what are other unanswered questions in the U.S. health reform debates?

It seems a primary question relates to *how* we are going to drastically lower healthcare spending in the next three to ten years. The risk is evident, that if we do not, healthcare spending will far exceed the ability of citizens to support the costs, either through tax dollars, insurance premiums or both.

With Social Security trustees alerting Americans and Congress for a second year in a row that Medicare is in serious trouble and the risk of unchecked spending is putting our Social Security reserves at risk, it seems evident that curtailing costs is the number one priority in any meaningful health reform effort. Health professionals understand that when bleeding is out of control, the hemorrhage must be stopped first. Any American who has withstood financial challenges knows that the first step is to *stop* spending. The process involves self-sacrifice, and tremendous discipline and endurance. Recovering from financial devastation is an incredibly intense, very painful process that requires self sacrifice and enormous hard work and sustained focus. But the pain does not last forever. And the benefits far exceed the expenditure of effort and energy.

These same "crisis management" skills will be needed in the long-term to restore balance and fiscal accountability to our healthcare system. A huge problem in previous efforts at health reform involves the enormous complexity of the U.S. healthcare system. There are so many large, powerful competing industries and lobbies, it's no wonder there is no money left for the poor patient, for whom the system was designed for in the first place.

A big issue will involve getting healthcare dollars realigned around the patient. And a big question for legislators is how they propose to achieve this.

More unanswered questions about healthcare stems from monies allocated for research. Currently, research on new medications is largely funded by pharmaceutical companies in the effort to bring the medications to market. Most prescription drugs brought to market—after initial testing for safety—are tested against placebos. Only occasionally are prescription drugs tested head-to-head, compared to each other or in comparison to another treatment. Rarely is CAM tested in comparison to pharmaceuticals.

For example, a new drug for high blood pressure is rarely tested against a blood pressure medicine that has been used for many years. And a new drug for high blood pressure is rarely, if ever, compared in its efficacy to a nonmedication solution, such as biofeedback, relaxation, yoga, or nutritional supplementation.

A great deal of anecdotal evidence shows that alternatives to medications can be helpful for people with chronic health challenges. Yet, substantial obstacles prevent their widespread use and implementation in conventional healthcare today. One is lack of money for quality research. Doctors and manufacturers in the CAM industry have not, had the revenue necessary for large-scale, quality scientific research.

At this point, the state of our nation's health remains dependent on the issue of funding. Who can afford research to document benefits of certain treatments and technologies? There may be effective CAM remedies, but no one will know about them because of lack of funds for available research. Perhaps if the American people feel strongly about the need for CAM research, a careful evaluation of federal research dollars will be done, and monies will be redirected toward CAM research. With trillions spent annually on U.S. healthcare, the crisis does not appear to be lack of funds, but rather the establishment of clear and specific directives for objective healthcare research.

What do the American people want? According to a recent article in *JAMA*, "The majority of Americans strongly support greater public and private funding for medical research."[167] "When asked what type of research was more valuable—disease prevention or cure—48 percent chose preventative research.[168] And "66 percent said the U.S. is spending too little on public health research, and 66 percent said at least twice as much should be spent."[169]

So a question to ask legislators is, who will pay to objectively research new health advances, regardless of ability to pay? This includes CAM products and services, as well as potentially beneficial conventional medicine therapies where a profit margin is not highly likely. For example, a specialized medication or surgery may exist that would likely benefit a small, specific number of patients, but the costs for development would likely far exceed any profits. Who would support such research financially and scientifically, in terms of product development?

Another important question to ask legislators is how they plan to remain objective about decisions regarding healthcare in cases where lobbies and special interest groups have supported the legislators financially. Also, how do legislators plan to engage in drastic cost containment with large, well-funded healthcare lobbies in Washington?

And how will the average American be able to actively participate in shaping a new model of healthcare?

And finally, how do legislators plan to drastically lower administrative and regulatory costs? How do they plan to create incentives for lower paying primary care physician careers? How do legislators plan to protect the health of American citizens against the onslaught of contaminants in air, water, soil, foods, and household products? How will the United States organize a collaborative effort in health transformation that includes environmental safety issues? How will people get the benefits of higher-priced technology only if and when they need it, while doing all that is possible to keep themselves healthy?

What, if any, would the role be of health savings accounts in a new healthcare system?

HSAs, approved in 2003, allow people to set aside money, tax-free, to pay for medical costs. Account holders must also have a health insurance policy with an annual deductible of at least $1,050 for individuals, $2,100 for a family.

Distributions may be tax-free if you use them to pay qualified medical expenses, which include:

- Obesity weight-loss programs
- Smoking cessation programs
- Immunizations
- Routine exams such as annual physicals
- Prenatal and well-child care
- Screening services to detect multiple conditions

Essentially, "medical care expenses include payments for the diagnosis, cure, mitigation, treatment or prevention of disease,"[170] including drugs; fees for doctors, dentists, surgeons, and chiropractors, as well as payments for hospital services, qualified long-term care services, nursing services, and laboratory fees.

Vitamins or nutritional supplements "do not count as qualified medical expenses unless they're recommended by

CHAPTER 11

A Twenty-First-Century Health Transformational Initiative

As we can see from the topics discussed in this book, health transformation is a complex topic, as complicated as healthcare itself. The purpose of this book is to make it all a little more understandable and lead you to more reading, study, discussion, and implementation.

It's obvious that the issue of CAM is still not widely discussed in the context of health reform. Yet it will likely be a true prescription for success in keeping patients healthier, lowering costs, and improving quality. What needs to happen in order for CAM to be integrated on a wide-spread level into conventional medicine? And what needs to take place in conventional healthcare to make room for CAM?

In *The Art of Transformation*, Gingrich and Desmond elaborate on transformational principles as America moves into the twenty-first century. They distinguish between reform and transformation: "Reform is a process of improving an existing system. Transformation is a method of visualizing a new system, culture, process, and structure, and migrating the current system to the new."[172] In reality, what we have been referring to as "health reform" is really the underpinnings of widescale health transformation. The two are very different.

Managed care represented massive health reform. A third-party, managed-care company was interposed between patients and their doctors. And until patients had received healthcare services, they were not even aware that a managed-care company was reviewing the health services rendered and had full authority to either authorize or deny the care.

Managed care was a service (or disservice, as many would say) interposed on top of the existing healthcare system. Other than the addition of managed care, including its additional layer of administration, the doctors, hospitals, and patients functioned in the same way.

What do we mean by transformation and how does this apply to healthcare? *The Art of Transformation* elaborates on seven key elements of a strategic plan for transformational change to take place:

1. Vision
2. Vision principles
3. Values
4. Metrics
5. Strategies
6. Projects
7. Habits[173]

Let us now apply these principles to U.S. health transformation to identify solutions to the current U.S. healthcare crisis.

Vision

The vision of a transformed U.S. health system is a healthy person. This can mean one of two objectives:

1. An individual who is able to remain disease-free by participating in the health strategies of the healthcare system
2. An individual whose health is restored as a direct result of his or her active participation in the healthcare system

Vision principles

All healthcare treatments and services in a transformed healthcare system are designed to promote and facilitate good health.

Principles include: prevention, safety, and cost-effectiveness available to all Americans. This include complementary and alternative modalities that have been tested scientifically and documented to be safe. Use of potentially risky interventions would be employed only when the safe ones are not enough to prevent disease. Riskier interventions would include medications and surgeries that have side effects as well as potential benefits. They would also include complementary and alternative therapies with potential side effects.

Medications have their place in a transformed healthcare system. They are not, however, the first line of promoting health and wellness. Medications are used cautiously and conservatively when the first lines of defense (CAM) have not been enough to prevent disease.

Many pharmaceutical companies are responding to the risks of side effects by developing medications that are much safer and easier for patients to tolerate. Some medications work incredibly well; others provide marginal benefits in relation to the cost to bring the drug to market and the costs to the consumer and the healthcare system.

In the current health system, neither doctors nor patients are given an opportunity to provide feedback on products and services that would be beneficial to patient care. I have little doubt that doctors and patients have incredible ideas to facilitate and promote our vision of health. In fact, CAM is full of such solutions. Until these ideas are tested on large numbers of patients in a standardized research setting, it is very difficult to determine which patients would benefit. Of course, CAM products do not carry the large profit margins to fund such research.

Can you envision a healthcare system in which doctors, at their monthly medical meetings, discussed and voted on the top ten priorities for healthcare research and development, and then submitted their results to a health advisory task force? And simultaneously, can you picture regular citizen forums to discuss and vote on upcoming research endeavors?

Of course, guidelines would need to adhere to our vision of health for all Americans. Technology proposals with no obvious health benefits but with large potential for profit automatically would be disqualified.

Values

The core value of a transformed healthcare system is the dignity and sanctity of life. This includes the inherent value of all people served in the health system and the lives of all the doctors and health professionals.

Replacing a piecemeal, bureaucratic, brutally competitive, antagonistic environment with the spirit of cooperation gives you a model that looks like this:

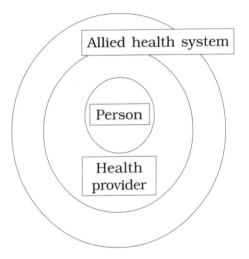

The transformed healthcare system has the individual at the center. This model is synergistic—everyone works together to help people get healthy and stay healthy. Notice the much smaller role of the allied health system, which includes all the indirect administrative healthcare costs. Its existence supports the health of the individual and the doctor's role in the individual's health.

Metrics

Metrics are a critical component of any health transformation efforts. Metrics represent that which is measurable. It is critical that research efforts measure health strategies that are helpful, safe, and cost-effective for any health transformation efforts to succeed. These include measuring conventional health strategies, CAM strategies, and integrative health strategies that combine both. Health outcomes, including quality-of-life data, are needed in all categories.

Similarly, cost-benefit analysis of integrative health strategies is needed to be compared with current conventional health costs.

Clearly, metrics will be indispensable in this transformation of health!

Strategies

Many strategies will transform U.S. healthcare in the upcoming decade:

- Demonstrating the safety and effectiveness of complementary and alternative medicine
- Demonstrating the safety and effectiveness of integrating conventional treatments with complementary and alternative ones
- Studying the long-term improvements in quality of life for healthy patients and patients with chronic health challenges treated with CAM and integrative health approaches
- Educating doctors on the results of research on complementary and alternative medicine
- Educating doctors on the results of research integrating conventional health with complementary and alternative medicine
- Educating patients on health choices based on quality, objective research
- Establishing quality standards of care based on the above research, while retaining the individual's freedom of choice
- Educating insurance companies on the results of the

above research, with subsequent implementation for an increase in patients' health choices to be covered by insurance

Projects

"Projects are the primary building blocks of change and the keys to implementing success.... Strategies at the highest level are broken down into projects."[174] Each of the above strategies has many defined projects. Many are research studies that will scientifically examine the potential benefits of complementary and alternative medicine choices. Many research projects will measure the potential benefits of integrative medicine for people with chronic health challenges.

In the past, our research in conventional healthcare has been haphazard and largely governed by profits. In a transformed healthcare system, our research projects will be recommended by doctors and educated citizens. Assigning monies and designating actual studies to various university research centers will be a serious and significant undertaking. Yet these are vital projects to design a transformed healthcare system. The successful completion of these research studies will establish standards of practice for patients that integrate conventional medicine with CAM.

Subsequent projects will include training physicians in integrative medicine and establishing holistic clinic models that are patient-friendly and easily replicable.

Many billions of administrative costs plague our conventional healthcare system. Part of the reason is the lack of uniformity and the massive expense to process so many diverse insurance plans and reimbursements. A transformational health system is simple—simple for patients and doctors to understand and simple and cost-effective to administer.

Another major project will be arriving at uniformity and simplicity with our insurance codes. As CAM becomes recognized and reimbursable by insurance companies, the need to simplify and standardize codes and methods will be essential.

Yet another major project will involve simplifying reimbursements. It would make sense to simplify each insurance provider's plans into three major plans: discount, intermediate, and premier. Then it would be standard and predictable to both the patient and provider what services are covered based upon what type of plan the patient has. Essentially, discount will function like an HMO, and the intermediate and premier like a PPO with an expanded selection of providers and services.

It remains to be decided how CAM will be reimbursed. This is a project in and of itself. CAM can be offered to varying degrees in the conventional plans—discount, intermediate, or premier; or it can be liberally reimbursed through health savings accounts. Regardless, the specifics of reimbursements for conventional and CAM procedures and treatments must be agreed upon and standardized in order to save the billions of dollars in administrative costs needed in this transformational healthcare system.

Other projects include establishing standards of training and licensing CAM professionals. Additional endeavors will include training conventional and CAM providers to work together and collaborate on patient care.

Habits

It seems intuitive that everyone involved in health transformation would engage in healthy life habits. This includes a proactive wellness commitment to life and modeling maturity and strength of character that participation in such transformational projects will take.

Every recommendation of the White House Commission on Complementary and Alternative Medicine Policy must be seen to completion. To achieve this and more, a Health Advisory Task Force must be appointed in Washington and challenged with the task of health transformation in this decade. The task force will consist of several task force subgroups:

1. Integrative Health Advisory Task Force: This group will bring together the most experienced physicians who know and understand how to integrate complementary and alternative health into mainstream medicine. Representatives of NCCAM must be included. The Integrative Health Advisory Task Force will examine the status of scientific research validating the use of natural supplements and natural modalities for two types of patients: healthy people trying to stay healthy and patients with chronic health challenges. Research studies must be conducted on the validity, safety, and effectiveness of various natural health modalities in helping improve the quality of life of patients who suffer from chronic diseases. The goal is to lessen their symptoms and possibly lower their doses of medications or possibly wean off medication altogether.

This subgroup will incorporate the results of doctors and citizens' votes on priorities for health research that are aligned with our vision of healthy people.

These studies will be conducted under the auspices of the Integrative Health Advisory Task Force and an independent Institutional Review Board to review the safety of research protocols. Such research could be conducted in quality U.S. medical training institutions as well as good private institutions. To remove any bias, no clinical investigator of such research studies will have any financial interests in any treatments or supplements offered in conventional or CAM systems.

These studies will also include large quality-of-life studies with significant numbers of healthy patients receiving natural supplements. The rates of illness or long-term health in these populations will be scrutinized over a period of at least five years. Such data will be instrumental in documenting the benefits—health-wise and cost-containment–wise—of natural health.

Along these lines, the FDA has prepared a draft document entitled "Evidence-Based Review of System for the Scientific Evaluation of Health Claims." Although a preliminary report, this document represents a promising start toward establishing guidelines for "an authorized health claim [that may be used] on both conventional foods and dietary supplements, provided that the substance in the product and the product itself meet the appropriate standards in the authorizing regulation."[175] The Integrative Health Advisory Task Force will amalgamate final FDA rulings with evidence-based claims for dietary supplements.

The task force will then make specific recommendations for the inclusion of complementary and alternative medicine into the mainstream healthcare system. These recommendations will be made first to the chair of the Health Advisory Task Force, and then to Congress as well as to the chief medical regulatory agencies, including the American Medical Association. These new integrative standards of care will be adopted, with continuing medical education courses offered to practicing physicians and an enhanced curriculum available for teaching medical students and residents.

After standards are established, widespread education for patients will take place in doctors' offices through video and teleconferencing.

The prescribed health model will empower patients to stay well and take charge of their health. Over time, the discussion of health responsibility will need to take place to address the issues of patient refusal to cooperate with a prescribed wellness plan.

2. Environmental Health Advisory Task Force: While this is happening, another subgroup of the Health Advisory Task Force needs to closely examine the issues of the environment and health, competing economic pressures, and realignment toward a healthier environment for all Americans. This Environmental Health Advisory Task Force will focus on creating a strategic plan to reduce environmental health challenges for all Americans in the next ten years. Representatives from the Environmental Protection Agency will be included. Discussion will include rating various products, services, and industries for their positive or negative impact on health. Following those determinations, the subgroup will outline consequences for products and services that are known to damage people's health. Also, members of this group will explore incentives to bring newer and safer technologies that are environment- and health-friendly. Recommendations of the Environmental Health Advisory Task Force will be presented to the chairman of the Health Advisory Task Force, then presented to and voted on by Congress.

3. Conventional Medicine Task Force: This subgroup of the Health Advisory Task Force will be commissioned to make recommendations to reform the current conventional healthcare system. This will include widespread reduction in bureaucracy, administrative, and regulatory costs. Health-reform leaders will be invited to speak and make suggestions, but the final recommendations will be made by the Conventional Medicine Task Force, presented to the chair of the Health Advisory Task Force and Congress, which will then vote on them. The mandate will be to lower the annual healthcare budget by billions of dollars that are currently spent on "indirect" or "nonpatient-related care."

This subgroup will also address the issues of profit incentives in healthcare. Economic incentives must include and encourage health-promoting industries and technologies. However, these businesses cannot unilaterally decide what healthcare and strategies are right for Americans and the U.S. healthcare system. Along these lines, this subgroup will decide how companies that want to introduce new scientific advances will submit bids for review prior to bringing new technologies to market. One criterion for selection must include affordability. It is recommended that health forums, including doctors and informed citizens, convene regularly.

The strategies outlined will effectively transform the practice of U.S. healthcare within the next five to seven years. If stalemates or irreparable disagreements in the subgroups occur, the unresolved issues may need to be brought to the American people for a vote. This health-transformation plan ultimately belongs to the people. Americans will need education on the various issues and a sense of empowerment before voting. Americans' responsibility will be to ensure that their constitutional rights are preserved in this new health plan. One of the synonyms for "healthy" is "full of life," so where there is health, there is life.

An essential component of our constitution's commitment to the life of Americans includes a fundamental commitment to keeping its citizens healthy. Health is much more than the absence of disease. The World Health Organization defines "health" as "a state of complete physical, mental, and social well-being and not merely the absence of disease or infirmity...healing necessarily includes a restoration of the inner resources of the spirit, and a connection to one's community and environment."[176]

In the same spirit of restoration, the principles behind health legislation must put people before profits.

CHAPTER 12

A Citizen's Role in Health Transformation

YOU HAVE LIKELY CONCLUDED BY NOW that transforming healthcare is a complex task, one that will take much time, effort, and attention from all Americans. Healthcare affects all of us, and it is incumbent on all of us to read, learn, and speak out in regard to important issues and decisions that will affect us and our families for years to come.

What else are we, as citizens, to do? We need to spend time listening and learning. We must make our voices heard. Then we need to educate others. Many of us have successfully integrated CAM into our conventional health-care treatments. We have done this by learning about complementary and alternative medicine on the Internet and in our pharmacies, and by consulting knowledgeable health practitioners. We've asked the right questions about the safety of natural health products used with conventional medicine. We are doing all we can do to stay well and healthy.

Now it is time to demand health and wellness from our legislators. When bills arise that support the use of complementary and alternative medicine, we must make our voices heard. We must get the word out in our communities. And while political debates are underway, we must let our legislators know that right now, they are only discussing half of the health-care equation. We must let them know when we've been helped by integrative health. We need to remind them that we have a right to get healthy and stay healthy. We deserve high-quality research documenting the safety and benefits of complementary and alternative medicine either alone or in combination with mainstream medicine. We need cost-effective preventative healthcare for ourselves and for our family. Yes, we have a right to be well and stay well.

We must remind our legislators that they voted for the creation of NCCAM—a division of NIH whose role and responsibility is to research quality complementary and alterative products and services and subsequently implement them into mainstream practice. We need to remind them that the final report of the White House Commission on Complementary and Alternative Medicine policy identifies many projects to prepare for this integration. We must again tell our legislators that the Environmental Protection Agency has many initiatives designed to promote and protect the health of all Americans; these initiatives need to be streamlined into the mainstream health-care system.

We cannot afford to be fooled by any statement by anyone who says health reform is easy. We need to understand that a system as complex as healthcare will not be transformed overnight. We must study and grasp the fundamental principles and stay active on legislative updates. Although the principles of health and wellness are simple, integrating them into conventional healthcare will be a complex process. It will take a lot of energy and concerted effort by doctors, patients, and health systems.

Let us all agree that all Americans need access to affordable healthcare.

Let us all agree that all Americans have the right to access the best preventative healthcare possible.

Let us all agree that any American with a health challenge has the right to access integrative health strategies that will help them get healthier and restore quality of life.

Let us *all* make a commitment to lower health-care costs while raising quality of health for all Americans.

The hope is that the concerted effort will be worthwhile, most of all for enhanced quality of life for American citizens, lowered health-care costs, and a commitment by all Americans to adopt health and wellness as a way of life.

Finally, let us all familiarize ourselves with the principles of The Good Health Plan. Let our efforts elaborate upon the principles but not diminish the integrity of their intent. The Good Health Plan is a health transformation proposal that offers drastically lowered health costs along with integrating complementary and alternative medicine for all Americans. The Good Health Plan takes the best of both conventional medicine and CAM and creates a new health-care system that is patient-centered and consumer-driven.

Lowered health costs are achieved by drastic simplification and standardization administratively, while investing in maintaining a healthy populus. In addition, citizen input and participation is vital, along with a streamlined health delivery system that is accessible, efficient, and affordable. By saving billions in excess administrative costs and system inefficiencies and by keeping people healthier, it is realistic that the current U.S. health-care budget not only stays fixed at $2 trillion but includes coverage for all Americans. The significance of this is simple yet profound: It will prevent the health-care industry from bankrupting our Social Security system and pave the way for meaningful reforms in other sectors of U.S. society.

It must be appreciated that creating a new health-care system will not happen overnight. In fact, while the U.S. healthcare system is in transition from an illness to a wellness model, it would be wise to view the health-care system as being "under construction." Thus, our thinking and reforms cannot be shortsighted or assume that a quick fix, person, or party will solve all the problems. For years, health-reform measures have failed because we have not taken a long-range strategy seriously enough. Also, the system has been very lucrative for some and has bankrupted others. The process of health transformation will take each and every one of us outside our comfort zone. With $2.3 trillion being spent *every year*, we, as Americans, must scrutinize where these dollars are going and learn to cut back and eliminate any and all dollars that are being spent wastefully.

The Good Health Plan provides a template—a roadmap, if you will—to drastically reduce bureaucratic inefficiencies and waste. We must scrutinize every dollar of spending as if it were our own. Between health insurance dollars and tax premiums, it is, after all, money spent by U.S. citizens that has funded and will continue to fund our healthcare. And with an aging baby boomer population, the dollars to invest in the system are dwindling, with current and projected expenditures clearly unsustainable.

Let's make our health-care system one of which we can be proud. One that will be there if we become ill and be there to lower our risk of getting sick in the first place. Let's be open to new strategies and services. Collectively, let's take responsibility for our health and make health transformation smooth and swift. The upcoming decade poses unprecendented challenges; a healthy America *will* be better equipped to handle them.

The Good Health Plan

A TRANSFORMED HEALTH SYSTEM REQUIRES new principles and practices. The Good Health Plan represents a healthcare proposal that incorporates the following principles:
1. Drastically lowering administrative/regulatory costs
2. Rewarding wellness and preventative medicine
3. Disease treatment that integrates complementary/ alternative medicine with mainstream conventional medicine
4. Incentives for patient-centered healthcare, including health forums and settings that are conducive to health, restoration, and healing with reduced costs

Ia. Managed care:
1. Automate all outpatient plan benefits/restrictions

2. Automate inpatient hospital plan benefits
   - When benefits are exceeded, case management specialist reviews care; either approves or denies care based on clinical Hx/Rx
   - After second hospitalization in one year, case management specialists automatically review cases with supervising physician; consideration of longer term care in a lower cost treatment setting; intensifying lower cost CAM products and services

Ib. Billing:
1. Simplify all insurance procedure codes:
   Current billing codes are currently based strictly on

diagnosis; over the next decade, care will include comprehensive stage-of-life care, in particular for health and wellness needs:

- Prenatal
- Child
- Adolescent
- Age 18–30
- Age 31–40
- Age 41–50
- Age 51–60
- Age 61–70
- Age 71–80
- Age 81–90
- Age 91 and over

Doctor visits will be categorized as wellness or illness:

- Individual Rx
- Group Rx
- Patient education
- Surgery and procedures

2. Consensus will be arrived at on three types of insurance plans, with standard rates and standard benefits that are predictable to the consumer (patient and family members) and health professionals. Thus, *all* health insurance plans will be simplified into:

- Plan A
- Plan B
- Plan C

Patients will have an insurance card to be used at the time of service, either office visit or hospital stay, with benefits clearly spelled out prior to the office visit or hospital stay.

In addition, catastrophic health coverage will be available now for all Americans. Catastrophic health plans are much less costly than standard plans, have very high deductibles (i.e., 10,000 per year) but cover medical catastrophes in amounts of 1 to 3 million dollars.

Also, health savings accounts, with high limits (5,000 to 10,000 dollars per year) should also be available to all

Americans. Complementary/alternative products and services should have unrestricted access, along with mainstream health services. In addition, health-promoting products such as organic fruits and vegetables should be covered under a health savings account.

During of the time the U.S. healthcare system is "under construction," the above will serve as stopgap measures to ensure no one is bankrupted by healthcare costs. In the next few years, after costs are drastically reduced and the health delivery system is enhanced greatly in its efficiency and ability to prevent illness, it is anticipated that a lowering of standard health insurance premiums will take place. So much so, that regardless of risk pools, health insurance should become affordable for the average American. This will dramatically improve quality of life for U.S. citizens, allowing job flexibility and the ability to switch from full- to part-time and will increase the opportunities for self- or home-based employment. In turn, this will reduce the incidence of stress-related illness in the workplace, thereby keeping our people healthier and more productive.

Ic. Regulatory:

Eliminate excess health delivery regulations that have arisen, largely, in response to the speed and depersonalization of our current healthcare system. These constitute regulations that take healthcare providers away from patient care, including excess paperwork.

However, increased regulations will take place for all vendors of products and nonprovider services in the healthcare industry. Items scrutinized will include ethics, conflicts of interest, and excess profits at patient and taxpayer expense. Health forums, which include citizens and health practitioners, will have the ability to report any suspected ethical violations with eventual hearings and decision making at the federal level. In addition, health insurance and vendor ethics will be monitored by the Health Advisory Task Force created in Washington and accountable to Congress and the American people. "Vendors" include manufacturers of pharmaceuticals, medical devices, technologies, and manufacturers of CAM products and services. Nonprovider services include those given in hospitals and outpatient clinics. The services include all nonmedical, including room and board and the like. Items to be scrutinized include salaries and fringe benefits of all nondirect patient care services.

II. Reward health and wellness:

People earn healthcare rebates—not based on diagnosis or preexisting conditions, but on how they follow their doctor's recommendations in all of the following areas:

- Physical—diet, exercise, health habits
- Mental—positive thinking, overcoming depression, anxiety, improved stress reduction
- Emotional—recovering from past abuse or trauma, moving from victim to empowerment; dealing in a healthy manner with anger and so forth
- Spiritual—deepening one's connection with a higher power

A person's progress is rated on an individualized, not the start point or the end point. In other words, if you are recovering from serious pain and trauma, you are not penalized; rather you are rewarded for the progress you are making.

An individual's productivity, or meaningful contribution to others, is also rated as a marker of health. With that, current laws restricting individuals who are disabled from working will be amended to encourage meaningful employment, taking disabilities and physical limitations into account.

III. Integration of complementary and alternative medicine into conventional healthcare with acceptance and implementation of recommendations in the White House Commission on Complementary and Alternative Medicine Policy:

A national committee of integrative health physicians with extensive clinical experience will develop a curriculum to commence widespread education of conventional healthcare providers.

Research on new and untested complementary and alternative medicine therapies will commence with results widely available to physicians and the public.

Simultaneously, the federal government will establish a Health Advisory Task Force that is accountable to Congress and the American people. The Health Advisory Task Force will consist of three subgroups:

1.Integrative Health Advisory Task Force: This will be composed primarily of physicians trained in both conventional and CAM, known as integrative health physicians. Requirements include primary responsibilities as based on clinical practice rather than primarily in research or education. Representatives of NCCAM are also included. As clinicians, their responsibilities will include:

- Establishing a database from integrative health practitioners of CAM and conventional medicine strategies that appear to be helpful in large numbers of patients.
- Listing potential side-effects of such strategies and the risks of not using such strategies.
- Examining clinical research data available in integrative medicine and identifying needs based on patient demand for further patient-centered research.
- Adoption of integrative medicine standards of practice for both management of illness and disease prevention. Such standards will be used to train physicians through continuing medical education and to medical students and residents. The standards for wellness and disease prevention will be adopted and utilized for stage-of-life community-based clinics.

2.Environmental Health Advisory Task Force: Will include physicians who specialize in environmental medicine, whose primary responsibility is caring for patients. Also included are members of the Environmental Protection Agency, along with professionals and citizens who are well versed in environmental health. Health practitioners with extensive knowledge of environmental health risk reduction must be included, such as naturopaths and CAM practitioners.

Responsibilities include making recommendations for products, services, and industries that promote health, while rating those that are at risk for causing or accelerating disease. Proposals for transitioning out of high-risk products and services to Americans will be made as well.

3. Conventional Medicine Task Force: This committee is tasked with the oversight and implementation of the recommendations to automate managed care, simplify insurance policies and premiums, and reduce health provider regulations. They should also be given the chance to recommend regulatory policies and procedures for the health insurance industry and nonprovider services. This task force will make recommendations to Congress to be voted on. Prior to making recommendations, the committee will hear reform proposals from the American Medical Association, the American Hospital Association, the health insurance industry, the managed care industry, and others.

In addition, the committee will study ways to offer incentives to primary care doctors and lower paid, high demand specialties and gradually lower costs and numbers of high-priced specialists and services. Recognizing this will take time, a gradual shift will occur in the next three to ten years. Study of the need for higher priced specialists when comprehensive health and wellness strategies are implemented will occur. Risks of high-priced technologies and surgeries will be further studied and placed in comparative clinical trials with lower priced health-promoting services. Long-term benefits of higher priced surgeries and technologies will be studied in specific-patient populations.

This committee will convene and collaborate with the Integrative Health Advisory Task Force, which will present models of care and training recommendations for primary care doctors who will now practice in an integrative health fashion.

IV. Patient-centered healthcare:

A. American citizens may not feel qualified to "drive" U.S. healthcare, but many are certainly qualified to actively participate in decisions driving health research and issues of spending allocations.

Regular health forums discussing potential studies and grants in major university settings will be held. Applicants for research dollars will present abstracts of potential studies with consumers voting on which studies best represent the public's priorities for directions in health research.

Up until now, citizens and patients have had no say in the directions of medical advances and new technologies. There has, up until now, been no fiscal accountability of the costs of new health advances to consumers, although ultimately, consumers are responsible for the costs of said advances.

The same process will take place with new pharmaceutical advances. Up until now, pharmaceutical companies have unilaterally determined what they believe are the most important areas for research and development. Now consumers will play an active role.

Citizens will also vote on complementary/alternative and integrative medicine directions for research.

Citizens who participate in such committees will be prescreened to ensure lack of bias and lack of financial incentives. Basic health knowledge will be expected of consumers in order to participate.

Health providers will also participate in such health forums and will likewise be prescreened for lack of financial incentives and lack of bias. These objective healthcare providers will vote on directives for research and new clinical advances in the practice of medicine.

The health forums will also review local healthcare spending and trends and will be empowered to make recommendations for changes in areas where spending seems disproportionate to the care that is given.

Local health forums will be accountable to a designated state health forum, which will represent findings on a national level.

B. As the American people get healthier, there will be reduced needs for acute-care hospital beds, which are incredibly costly. Yet, people who are recovering from illness may need longer time with medically supervised care that does not meet the acuity of a hospital ward. In time, vacant hospital wards could be converted to longer term recovery/rehabilitation units. Particularly with the rising numbers of aging baby boomers, this new, less expensive model of recovery will likely become very popular and much more cost-effective.

C. To lower the pressure on emergency rooms, urgent care settings that handle lower acuity health issues should be widespread and located in close proximity to emergency rooms. Many people who walk into emergency rooms could be handled very effectively and at lower cost in an urgent care setting. Patients could be triaged by a nurse who could direct patients to either the emergency room or urgent care walk-in clinic, depending on the severity of their condition. Typically, urgent care settings are open reduced hours, but they could be open around the clock to treat health issues promptly in a more cost-effective manner.

D. Electronic health records will contribute considerably to improved patient care at lowered costs, particularly in the urgent care and emergency room settings, by instant accessibility to a patient's laboratory and other diagnostic tests. Too often, those tests are repeated regularly, causing patient inconvenience and markedly excess costs. Electronic health records will also save lives by having built-in alarms at the slightest detection of a drug-drug interaction or a critical lab value posing a potentially life-threatening crisis.

E. Twenty-four-hour pharmacies will also provide an indispensable resource to alert patients of potential drug-drug interactions and drug-herb interactions. As CAM becomes integrated into mainstream healthcare, such up-to-date information will be a vital resource for both patients and healthcare providers.

F. Incentives must exist for medical students to pursue primary care/family practice and specialties that relate to direct, front-line patient care, such as pediatrics, ob-gyn, and behavioral health. In many areas of the United States, there exists a critical shortage of these practitioners, thus increasing health risks to citizens. Training will include integration of CAM into mainstream medicine.

This will also require stabilizing doctor reimbursement as well as encouraging doctors to work in clinics, offices, and walk-in clinics. Eventually, integrative health doctors will serve as consultants to the stage-of-life clinics.

As stated earlier, the study and implementation of these incentives and the development of the stage-of-life clinics will occur primarily with the Integrative Health Advisory

Task Force.

G. Because stage-of-life clinics will offer classes and services in community settings, overhead costs will be much lower. Patients can be seen for routine wellness and preventative care in places that are convenient, so health and wellness is routinely integrated into their day. Participation in these preventative wellness classes will be rewarded by improved health and lowered health insurance premiums. Stage-of-life clinics may be located in other community settings such as churches, adult education institutions, civic centers, and athletic centers. Standards will be set nationally with results achieved locally. As reimbursement details are finalized, these centers will be given a stipend for hosting the stage-of-life clinics.

Bibliography

ADD Health and Wellness Centers Inc. Addison, TX. http://www.addhealthandwellness.com (accessed September 10, 2007).

Alliance for Health Reform. "Employer Retirement Income Security Act (ERISA) and State Health Reform." Alliance for Health Reform (August 10, 2007).

Alternative Health Insurance Services. "Health Savings Accounts." http://www.althlthins.com/html/health savings.htm (accessed November 26, 2007).

Alvarez, R, MD and M. Murakami. "What Doctors Should Know about CAM." June 2003. Chi Fountain Integrative Medicine. San Francisco: http://www.chifountain.com (accessed November 25, 2007).

American Academy of Pediatrics. "Counseling Families Who Choose Complementary psychological support to resolve past issues, including trauma, would seem to go along way to and Alternative Medicine for their Child With Chronic Illness or Disability." *Pediatrics* 107, No. 3 (March 2001): 598–601.

American Academy of Environmental Medicine. http://www.aaem.com (accessed September 8, 2008); http://www.aaem.com/education.html

American Hospital Association. "Protecting and Improving Care for Patients and Communities, Coordinating Care for the Chronically Ill." American Hospital Association, Annual Meeting Coordinating Care for the Chronically Ill, May 1, 2005.

American Institute of Stress. "America's No.1 Health Problem." American Institute of Stress. http://www.stress.org/americas.htm (accessed September 2, 2007).

American Institute of Stress. "Job Stress," www.stress.org/job.htm.

American Medical Association. "Medical Student Debt." American Medical Association. http://www.ama-assn.org (accessed December 9, 2007).

Astin, John A. "Why Patients Use Alternative Medicine." Journal of the American Medical Association 279, no. 19 (May 20, 1998): 1,548–1,553.

Baker, Fraser L., PhD. http://www.CAM-Admin.com, "Complementary and Alternative Medicine Explained" 2007 (accessed February 9, 2008).

Barnes, P., Powell-Griner,E., McFann,K, and Nahin R.. "Complementary and Alternative Medicine Use Among Adults: United States, 2002": Advance Data, Centers for Disease Control and Prevention No. 343 (May 27, 2004).

Begany, Timothy. "Alternative Medicine: Is It Viable in Asthma and Allergy?" Respiratory Reviews 8, no. 1 (January 2003).

The Blair McGill & Hill Advisory. "Top 10 Steps to Protect Your Assets: Increasing Litigation." The Blair, McGill & Hill Group, LLC (2000): NewSmile.com (accessed November 22, 2007).

Brown, V., J. Grootjans, J. Ritchie, M. Townsend, and G. Verrinder. "Sustainability and Health, Supporting Global Ecological Integrity in Public Health." Earthscan (2005): London, Sterling, VA.

Burton Report. "Utilization Review." http://www. burtonreport.com (accessed December 8, 2007).

California Healthline. "Study: Health Care for Iraq Veterans Could Exceed $650 Billion." California Healthline (November 9, 2007).

CAM at the National Institutes of Health. *Focus on Complementary and Alternative Medicine* XIV, No. 3 (Summer 2007). http://nccam.nih.gov/news/newsletter/2007_summer/ stakeholders.htm.

Centers for Disease Control and Prevention National Center for Health Statistics. http://www.cdc.gov/nchs/ fastats/overwt.htm (accessed February 1, 2008).

————. "Complementary and Alternative Medicine Use Among Adults: United States, 2002." Advance Data From Vital and Health Statistics no. 343 (May 27, 2004).

CDC National Institute for Occupational Safety and Health. *NIOSH Publication No. 99–101*. http://www.cdc.gov/niosh/ stresswk.html (accessed September 4, 2007).

Centers for Medicare and Medicaid Services. "National Health Expenditure Data." "National Health Expenditure Projections 2006–2016." U.S. Department of Health and Human Services. http://www.cms.hhs.gov/ NationalHealthExpendData/downloads/proj2006.pdf (accessed September 6, 2007).

The Center for Mind-Body Medicine. http://www.cmbm.org (accessed September 5, 2007). About Us: http:// www.cmbm.org/mind_ body_medicine_ABOUT/ about_center_for_mind_ body_medicine_cmbm.php

Collaborative on Health and the Environment Toxicant and Disease Database. "The Collaborative on Health and the Environment." http://database.healthand environment. org (accessed November 26, 2007).

Consumer Affairs. "Many Young Adults Lack Health Insur-

ance." Consumer Affairs, (May 24, 2006) http://
www.printthisclickability.com (accessed December 7, 2007).

Conover, Christopher, J. "Health Care Regulation A $169
Billion Hidden Tax." *Policy Analysis*, Cato Institute, no.
527 (October 4, 2004).

Corbett Clark, Mary, "The Cost of Job Stress." *Winning Workplaces*. http://www.winningworkplaces.org/library/fea-
tures/the_cost_of_job_stress.php (accessed November 11,
2007).

Croen, LA, Najjar,D., Ray,T. et al. "A Comparison of Health
Care Utilization and Costs of Children With and Without
Autism Spectrum Disorders in a Large Group Model
Health Plan." *Pediatrics* Vol. 118,No.4,October 2006.

Davidoff, A. and G. Kenney. "Uninsured Americans with
Chronic Health Conditions." *Urban Institute* (May 2, 2005).

DeVol, R. and A. Bedroussian "An Unhealthy America: The
Economic Burden of Chronic Disease—Charting a New
Course to Save Lives and Increase Productivity and Eco-
nomic Growth." The Milken Institute (October 2007).

Eisenberg, D., Kessler, R., Foster, C., Norlock, F., Calkins,
D. and Delbanco, T., "Unconventional Medicine in the
United States—Prevalence, Costs, and Patterns of Use."
New England Journal of Medicine 328 (January 28,
1993),Number 4: 246–252.

Environmental Defense, "About Us>>Mission Statement";
http://www.environmentaldefense.org (accessed December 8, 2007).

Environmental Defense. "Asthma, Traffic and Air Pollution" Environmental Defense (updated August 8, 2007) http://
www.environmentaldefense.org (accessed December 8, 2007).

Environmental Defense. "Cleaning Up Dirty School Buses."
(November 8, 2007) http://www.environmental
defense.org (accessed December 8, 2007).

———. "What Will Global Warming Inaction Cost? The Financial Burdens of Doing Nothing Explained." Environmental Defense. (November 14, 2007) http://www.environmentaldefense.org (accessed December 8, 2007).

——— "The Science: Increased Health Risks of Traffic." Environmental Defense (April 19, 2007). http://www.environmentaldefense.org (accessed December 8, 2007).

Families USA. "Why Insurance Matters." (June 2004) quoting K. Davis *Time for Change: The Hidden Cost of a Fragmented Health Insurance System* New York: The Commonwealth Fund, 2003.

Gabriel, Gerald, "Hans Seyle: The Discovery of Stress", www.brainconnection.com (accessed March 15, 2008).

Gay, L. "Fruits, vegetables not as nutritious as 50 years ago." *Seattle Post-Intelligencer*, Scripps Howard News Service. (March 1, 2006).

Gingrich, N., and N. Desmond. *The Art of Transformation.* Washington, D.C., CHT Press, 2006.

Goodman, J., G. Musgrave, and D. Herrick. *Lives at Risk.* Lanham, MD: Rowman & Littlefield Publishers, 2004.

Gratzer, D. *The Cure.* New York: Encounter Books, 2006.

Health News. "Americans Want Stronger Commitment to Health Research." *Daily News Central.* (September 21, 2005).

———. "Healthcare Costs to Account for 20% Economy." *Daily News Central.* (February 23, 2006).

———. Herbert, Martha, MD, PhD. "Time to Get a Grip." *Autism Advocate*, 5th ed., 2006.

Herzlinger, R., PhD, ed. *Consumer-Driven Health Care Implica-*

tions for Providers, Payers and Policy Makers. Wiley and Sons, April 2004.

Hileman, Bette, "Children's Health is Declining, Says American Chemical Society." http://www.antibiotic-alternatives.com/childrens_health.htm (accessed September 12, 2007).

Hitti, Miranda. "CDC: 1 in 150 Kids May Have Autism." (February 8, 2007) http://www.MedicineNet.com (accessed September 5, 2007).

Huerta E. Testimony before the WHCCAMP. March 26, 2001; in White House Commission on Complementary and Alternative Medicine Policy Final Report. U.S. Government Printing Office (March 2002) http://bookstore.gpo.gov.

Institute for Functional Medicine, http://www.functionalmedicine.org; http://www.functional medicine.org/about/mission.asp; http://www.functional medicine.org/about/whatis.asp.

Institute of Medicine. "Care Without Coverage Too Little Too Late." Institute of Medicine. (May 2002).

JAMA and Archives Journals (2007, April 3). Autism Costs Society An Estimated $3 Million Per Patient, According To Report. *ScienceDaily.* Retrieved March 15, 2008, from http://www.sciencedaily.com-/releases/2007/04/070403112757.htm.

Jones, David, MD, Editor in Chief. *Textbook of Functional Medicine.* Gig Harbor, WA: Institute for Functional Medicine, 2005.

Kaiser Commission on Medicaid and the Uninsured. "The Cost of Not Covering the Uninsured." (June 2003).

Kaiser Daily Health Policy Report. "Health Insurance Claims Denials Cost Billions in Administrative Costs." Kaiser Network. (February 16, 2007) http://www.kaisernetwork.org (accessed September 5, 2007).

———. "White, Middle-Age Americans in Worse Health than British Counterparts, Despite Higher U.S. Health Care Spending." Kaiser Network. (May 3, 2006) http://www.kaisernetwork.org (accessed September 2, 2007).

———. "Women's Health: Comprehensive Study Calls U.S. Policy and Status 'Unsatisfactory.'" Kaiser Network. (August 23, 2000) http://www.kaisernetwork.org (accessed September 14, 2007).

Kaiser Family Foundation. "How Changes in Medical Technology Affect Health Care Costs." Kaiser Family Foundation. (March 2007) http://www.kff.org (accessed September 2, 2007).

———. "Snapshots: Health Care Costs: Health Care Spending in the United States and OECD Countries." Kaiser Family Foundation. (January 2007) http://www.kff.org (accessed September 2, 2007).

———. "The Uninsured: A Primer, Key Facts About Americans without Health Insurance." Kaiser Family Foundation. (October 2007).

———. "Trends in Health Care Costs and Spending". Kaiser Family Foundation (September 2007); http://www.kff.org (accessed March 16, 2008).

Kendall, D., Tremain, K, Lemieux, J and Levine, S.R. "Healthy Aging v. Chronic Illness: Preparing Medicare for the New Health Challenge." Global Action on Aging (February 14, 2003).

Kligler, B., MD, MPH, and R. Lee, MD. *Integrative Medicine Principles for Practice*. United States, McGraw Hill, Medical Publishing Division, 2004.

Kling, A. *Crisis of Abundance*. Washington, DC: Cato Institute, 2006.

Lee, Phillip, R., MD. "Welcome, The Collaboration on Health and the Environment," http://www.healthand

environment.org (accessed March 12, 2008).

Lee, R. and R. Edwards. "The Fiscal Impact of Population Aging in the U.S.: Assessing the Uncertainties." Center for the Economics and Demography of Aging, Institute of Business and Economics Research (2002).

MacWilliam, Lyle, MSc, FP. *Nutrisearch Comparative Guide to Nutritional Supplements.* 4th ed. United States of America, Northern Dimensions Publishing, 2007.

Mahar, Maggie. *Money Driven Medicine, The Real Reason Health Care Costs So Much.* New York: Harper Collins, 2005.

Managed Care Resources. "Managed Care Terms and Definitions." Managed Care Resources. http://www.mcres.com (accessed December 8, 2007).

Marcotte, D., V. Wilcox-Gok, and P. Redmon. "Prevalence and Patterns of Major Depressive Disorder in the United States Labor Force." *The Journal of Mental Health Policy and Economics* 2, 123–131(1999).

Mayo Foundation for Medical Education and Research. "Chronic Stress: Can it cause depression?" Mayo Foundation for Medical Education and Research. http://www.mayoclinic.com/health/stress/AN1286 (accessed December 1, 2007).

———. "Complementary and Alternative Medicine: What is it?" Mayo Foundation for Medical Education and Research. (October 26, 2007) http://www.nlm.nih.gov/medlineplus/complementaryand alternativemedicine.html, (accessed December 9, 2007).

McLean, Thomas R. and Richards, Edward P., "Health Care's "Thirty Years War": The Origins and Dissolution of Managed Care." *NYU Annual Survey of American Law* 60, June 4, 2004; 283–328.

Medical News Today. "Mankind is Predisposed to Diseases of Civilization." (August 27, 2005) http://

www.medicalnewstoday.com (accessed January 26, 2008).

Michigan in Brief. "Health Care Costs and Managed Care." Michigan in Brief. (April 1, 2002) 5; http:// www.michiganinbrief.org (accessed October 22, 2007).

Mercola.com. "Healthy Fast Food is No Better for Your Heart" *The American Journal of Clinical Nutrition* 862 (August 2007): 334–340.

Mock, Geoffrey. "Is Excessive Health Care Regulation Hurting Uninsured?" Duke University, News and Communications, February 9, 2004.

Mokdad, A. H., J. S. Marks, et al. "Actual Causes of Death in the United States, 2000." *JAMA* 291 (2004): 1,238–1,245.

MSNBC.com, "Report: 35 percent of toys contain lead." Associated Press, December 4, 2007. http:// www.msnbc.msn.com/id/22103641/ (accessed December 5, 2007).

National Center for Complementary and Alternative Medicine, National Institutes of Health. http:// www.nccam.nih.gov (accessed September 6, 2007): "What is CAM", http://nccam.nih.gov/health/whatiscam (accessed March 15, 2008). NCCAM Facts-at-a-Glance and Mission, http://nccam.nih.gov/about/ataglance.

National Environmental Health Association. "Children's Environmental Health." National Environmental Health Association (July 2, 1997) http://www.neha.org/ position_papers/PositionChildren.html (accessed September 12, 2007).

National Public Radio. "New Emphasis on Doctor-Patient Relations." National Public Radio (October 6, 2003) http:/ /www.npr.org (accessed October 25, 2007).

Proctor, Jennifer. "Treating Physician's Career Woes." *AAMC Reporter* 9, no. 10 (July 2000), p.1–5.

Quattrini, S. "The Decline in the Patient-Physician Relationship." http://www.albany.edu (accessed November 22, 2007).

Rich, Deborah. "Organic Fruits and Vegetables Work Harder for Their Nutrients." San Francisco (March 25, 2006) http://gate.com (accessed December 8, 2007).

Rogers, Sherry, MD. *Detoxify or Die.* Florida: Sand Key Company, 2002.

Rona, Zoltan, MD. "Childhood Illness and the Allergy Connection." http://www.all-natural.com (accessed November 24, 2007).

Rosner, David. "US History Companion, Medicine." http://www.answers.com (accessed December 9, 2007).

SafesourceRx.com. "US: facing aging population challenges as 77M US Boomers near retirement age." (2007) http://www.safesourcerx.com/articles/aging/agingTrends.asp (accessed December 5, 2007).

SAMHSA. "Alternative Approaches to Mental Health Care." National Mental Health Information Center, United States Department of Health and Human Services. http://mentalhealth.samhsa.gov/publications (accessed November 17, 2007).

Sawyer-Morse, Mary Kaye, PhD, RD. "What's for Dinner? Factors that Influence Food Choices." *Today's Dietician* 7, No. 10 Vol.7, 68; http://www.todaysdietician.com/newachives/td_1005p68.shtml (accessed December 8, 2007).

Starfield, B., MD. "America's Healthcare System is the Third Leading Cause of Death." Summary by Kah Ying Choo. *JAMA* 284 no. 4 (July 26, 2000): 483–485. http://www.health-care-reform.net/causedeath.htm (accessed December 8, 2007).

Thomasson, M. "Health Insurance in the United States."

EH Net*Encyclopedia* http://thomasson.insurance. health.us (accessed December 7, 2007).

"U.S. Autism Rates Rise Sharply." Health Day News, Monday, March 7, 2005; http://www.ajc.com/health/content/shared-auto/healthnews/kids/524376.html (accessed September 12, 2007).

U.S. Environmental Protection Agency. "Draft Report on the Environment 2003." U.S. Environmental Protection Agency. http://www.epa.gov (accessed January 26, 2008).

———. "Sustainability Basic Information." (August 20, 2007) U.S. Environmental Protection Agency. http:// www.epa.gov/sustainability/basicinfo.htm (accessed January 29, 2008).

U.S. Food and Drug Administration. "Guidance for Industry, Evidence-Based Review System for the Scientific Evaluation of Health Claims, Draft Guidance." U.S. Food and Drug Administration, Center for Food Safety and Applied Nutrition (July 2007).

Wang, Stewart C. "An Aging Population: Fragile, Handle with Care." NHTS People Saving People, Ciren Aging Population, http://www-nrd.nhtsa.dot.gov/departments/nrd-50/ciren/um_fragile.html (accessed December 5, 2007).

WebMD. "Depression Linked to Parkinson's" reviewed by Gary D. Vogin, MD, Parkinson's Disease Health Center (May 28, 2002) http://www.WebMD.com (accessed September 4, 2007).

Weil, Andrew, MD. http://www.integrativemedicine. arizona.edu (accessed February 9, 2008); http:// www.integrativemedicine.arizona.edu/about2.html; http://www.integrativemedicine.arizona.edu/ about2.html#principles; http://www.integrativemedicine. arizona.edu/af/index.html.

White House Commission on Complementary and Alternative Medicine Policy. Final Report. U.S. Government

Printing Office (March 2002) http://bookstore.gpo.gov.

Winslow, Lisa Corbin and Howard Shapiro. "Physicians Want Education About Complementary and Alternative Medicine to Enhance Communication With Their Patients." *Archives of Internal Medicine* 162 (2002): 1,176–1,181.

Wright, Jonathan. "Fruits and Vegetables May Lack Nutrient Content." http://www.wrightnewsletter.com/etips/ht200502/ht20050224.html (accessed December 8, 2007).

World Health Organization. "An estimation of the economic impact of chronic noncommunicable diseases in selected countries." Department of Chronic Diseases and Health Promotion (2006).

———. "Preventing Disease Through Healthy Environments, Towards an estimate of the environmental burden of disease" (2006).

———. *The World Health Report 2000-Health Systems: Improving Performance*. World Health Organization, Geneva, Switzerland.

Zimm, A. "Chronic Illnesses on Rise." *Bloomberg News* (June 27, 2007) http://boston.com (accessed January 26, 2008).

Zwillich, T. "U.S. Not Ready for Rise in Disabled." WebMD Health News (April 24, 2007) http://www.WebMD.com (accessed December 7, 2007).

Notes

[1] Kaiser Family Foundation, "Snapshots: Health Care Costs," 1.
[2] Health News, "Healthcare Costs to Account for 20% Economy," 1.
[3] http://nccam.nih.gov/health/whatiscam
[4] White House, Final Report, 7
[5] Barnes et al., "Complementary and Alternative Use Among Adults," 1.
[6] Ibid., 1.
[7] White House, Final Report,xvii.
[8] Eisenberg, "Unconventional Medicine," 1.
[9] Winslow, "Physicians Want Education", 1.
[10] Kaiser Family Foundation, "Snapshots: Health Care Costs," 1.
[11] Kaiser Family Foundation, "Trends in Health Care Costs and Spending",1.
[12] Centers for Medicare and Medicaid Services, "National Health Expenditure Data",1.
[13] Kaiser Family Foundation, "The Uninsured," 1.
[14] Ibid., 1.
[15] The World Health Report 2000-Health Systems: Improving Performance, XX.
[16] Thomasson, "Health Insurance in the United States," 1.
[17] Ibid., 3.
[18] Ibid,3.
[19] Ibid.3.
[20] Ibid., 4.
[21] McLean and Richards, "Health Care's 'Thirty Years War,'" 285.

22 Ibid., 287.
23 Thomasson, "Health Insurance in the United States," 6.
24 Managed Care Resources, "Managed Care Terms and Definitions," 16.
25 Ibid., 31.
26 Proctor, "Treating Physician's Career Woes," 1,2.
27Kaiser Network, "Insurance Claims Denials", 1
28 Burton Report, "Utilization Review," 1.
29 Blair McGill & Hill Advisory, "Steps to Protect Your Assets," 1.
30 Kaiser Network, "Insurance Claims Denials", 1.
31Ibid., 1.
32 Kaiser Family Foundation, "The Uninsured," 1.
33 Ibid.,1.
34 Davidoff,A.and Kenney,G., "Uninsured Americans with Chronic Health Conditions",1.
35 Institute of Medicine, "Care Without Coverage," 1.
36 Ibid., 1.
37 Ibid., 1.
38 Families USA, "Why Insurance Matters," 2.
39 Institute of Medicine, "Care Without Coverage," 5.
40 Consumer Affairs, "Young Adults Lack Insurance," 1.
41 Ibid., 1.
42 Kaiser Commission, "Cost of Not Covering the Uninsured," 3.
43 World Health Report 2000, "Health Systems: Improving Performance," 152.
44 Kaiser Family Foundation, "Changes in Medical Technology," 1.
45 Ibid., 1.
46 Mahar, "Money Driven Medicine," xviii.
47 American Medical Association, "Medical Student Debt," 2.
48 Rosner, "US History Companion, Medicine," 3.
49 Conover, "Health Care Regulation," 1.
50 Mock, "Health Care Regulation Hurting Uninsured?" 1.
51 Ibid., 2.
52 Conover, "Health Care Regulation," 1.
53 Ibid., 1.
54 DeVol et al., "An Unhealthy America," i.
55 Ibid., ii.
56 Ibid., 1.
57 Ibid., i.

[58] Ibid., 2.

[59] American Hospital Association, "Protecting and Improving Care," 1.

[60] Ibid., 1.

[61] Kaiser Daily Health Policy Report, "Women's Health," 1.

[62] Kaiser Daily Health Policy Report, "Americans in Worse Health than British," 1.

[63] Ibid., 1.

[64] Ibid., 1.

[65] American Institute of Stress, "America's No.1 Health Problem" ,1.

[66] Gabriel, Gerald, "Hans Seyle: The Discovery of Stress",1.

[67] American Institute of Stress, "Stress,America's No.1 Health Problem" 1.

[68]American Institute of Stress, "Job Stress",1..

[69] CDC, NIOSH Publication No. 99–101, 2.

[70] Corbett Clark, "The Cost of Job Stress," 2.

[71] Mayo Foundation, "Chronic Stress," 1.

[72] Marcotte, Wilcox-Gok, and Redmon, "Prevalence of Major Depressive Disorder," 125.

[73] WebMD, "Depression Linked to Parkinson's," 1.

[74] Rich, "Organic Fruits and vegetables," 1.

[75] Rich, "Organic Fruits and vegetables," 1.

[76] Sawyer-Morse, "What's for Dinner?" 1.

[77] Medical News Today, "Mankind is Predisposed to Diseases," 1.

[78] Zimm, "Chronic Illnesses on Rise," 1.

[79] Ibid,1.

[80] Ibid, 1.

[81] Centers for Disease Control and Prevention National Center for Health Statistics, 1.

[82] Mercola.com, "Healthy Fast Food," 1.

[83] Ibid., 1.

[84] Rich, "Organic Fruits and Vegetables,"2.

[85] Rich, "Organic Fruits and vegetables,"2.

[86] Wright, "Fruits and Vegetables May Lack," 1.

[87] Lee and Edwards, "Fiscal Impact of Population Aging," 4.

[88] SafesourceRx.com, "US: facing challenges," 1.

[89] Lee and Edwards, "Fiscal Impact of Population Aging," Abstract.

[90] Kendall et al., "Healthy Aging v. Chronic Illness," 1.

[91] Ibid., 2.

[92] Mokdad et al., "Actual Causes of Death," XX.

[93] SafesourceRx.com, "US: facing challenges," 1.
[94] Ibid., 1.
[95] Ibid., 2.
[96] Ibid., 2.
[97] Ibid., 3.
[98] Wang, "An Aging Population," 1.
[99] Ibid., 1.
[100] Zwillich, "U.S. Not Ready," 1.
[101] Ibid., 1.
[102] California Healthline, "Health Care for Iraq Veterans," 1.
[103] World Health Organization, "Preventing Disease," 5.
[104] EPA, "Draft Report on the Environment 2003," 4–10.
[105] Lee, "The Collaboration on Health and the Environment" 1.
[106] Ibid,1.
[107] Rogers, *Detoxify or Die*, 159.
[108] Ibid., 167.
[109] Ibid., 162.
[110] Hileman, "Children's Health is Declining," 1.
[111] National Environmental Health Association, "Children's Environmental Health," 1.
[112] Ibid., 2.
[113] Hileman, "Children's Health is Declining," 1.
[114] Ibid., 1.
[115] Herbert, "Time to Get a Grip," 19.
[116] Ibid., 21.
[117] Croen et al., "A Comparison of health care utilization," 2.
[118] JAMA and Archives Journals(2007, April3) Autism Costs Society...1.
[119] "U.S. Autism Rates Rise," 1.
[120] MSNBC.com, "Toys contain lead," 1.
[121] U.S. EPA, "Sustainability Basic Information," 1.
[122] Ibid.1.
[123] Brown et al, "Sustainability and Health," 3.
[124] Environmental Defense, About Us>>Mission Statement,1.
[125] Ibid,1.
[126] Environmental Defense, "Global Warming Inaction Cost?," 2.
[127] Environmental Defense, "Cleaning Up Dirty School Buses," 1.

128 Environmental Defense, "Asthma, Traffic and Air Pollution," 1.
129 Environmental Defense,"The Science:Increased Health Risks of Traffic,1.
130 Kligler and Lee, *Integrative Medicine Principles*, 3.
131 Starfield, "America's Healthcare System," 2.
132 Quattrini, "Decline in the Patient-Physician Relationship," 1.
133 NPR, "Emphasis on Doctor-Patient Relations," 1.
134 Herzlinger, *Consumer-Driven Health Care Implications*, XX.
135 Ibid., XX.
136 National Center for Complementary and Alternative Medicine, 1.
137 CDC; Complementary and Alternative Medicine Use Among Adults,1.
138 White House, Final Report, 7..
139 National Center for Complementary and Alternative Medicine, 'What is CAM?",1.
140 Alvarez & Murakami, "What Doctors Should Know About CAM",1.
141 SAMHSA, "Alternative Approaches to Mental Health Care," 1.
142 White House, Final Report, 11.
143 Huerta E. Testimony before the WHCCAMP,1.
144 Astin, "Why Patients Use Alternative Medicine," 2.
145 American Academy of Pediatrics, "Counseling Families," 2.
146 Rona, Zoltan, MD. "Childhood Illness and the Allergy Connection
147 Baker, Fraser L., PhD. http://www.CAM-Admin.com
148 Begany, Timothy, "Alternative Medicine: Is it Viable in Asthma and Allergy?"1.
149 http://www.functionalmedicine.org/about/mission.asp
150 http://www.functionalmedicine.org/about/whatis.asp
151 http://www.integrativemedicine.arizona.edu/about2.html
152 http://www.integrativemedicine.arizona.edu/about2.html#principles
153 http://www.integrativemedicine.edu/af/index.html
154 http://www.aaem.com
155 http://www.aaem.com/education.html
156 NCCAM, "What is CAM?" http://nccam.nih.gov/health/whatiscam

[157] CAM at the NIH,Focus on Complementary and Alternative Medicine, http://nccam.nih.gov/news/newsletter/2007_summer/stakeholders.htm,1.

[158] Ibid,1.

[159] Center for Mind Body Medicine, http://www.cmbm.org/mind_body_medicine_ABOUT/about_center_for_mind_body_medicine_cmbm.php

[160] White House Commission, xviii.

[161] Goodman,Musgrave,Herrick, "Lives at Risk," 11.

[162] Ibid., 18.

[163] Ibid., 17.

[164] Ibid., 70.

[165] Ibid., 34.

[166] Ibid., 177.

[167] Health News, "Americans Want Stronger Commitment,"1.

[168] Ibid., 2.

[169] Ibid., 2.

[170] Alternative Health Insurance Services, "Health Savings Accounts," 2.

[171] Ibid., 2.

[172] Gingrich and Desmond, *The Art of Transformation*, 7.

[173] Ibid., 111–123.

[174] Ibid., 134.

[175] U.S. Food and Drug Administration. "Guidance for Review System," 3.

[176] Klinger and Lee, Integrative Medicine Principles, 11.

Index

Food and Drug
Administration (*see*
FDA)
food supply, abundance of
U.S., 31
food, organic, and benefits
from eating, 33–34, 101

Ganz, Michael, 42–43
Global Action on Aging, 35
Good Health Plan, the, 97–
98, 99–107
and billing in, 99–101
and the Conventional
Medicine Task Force in,
104
and the Environmental
Health Advisory Task
Force in, 103–104
and the Integrative Health
Advisory Task Force in,
103
and integration of CAM in,
102–103
and managed care, 99
and patient-centered
health care in, 104–107
and regulations in, 101–102
and wellness rewarded in,
102
Gordon, James S., 72
Great Depression, the, 9
gross national product, 7

Haldol, 24
health care:
citizen role in transformed
system of, 95–98
evolution of current system,
9–11
and high cost of premiums,
8
importance of healthy
habits in transformed
system of, 89–93

key elements for
transformational change
of, 84–93
metrics of transformed
system of, 87
principles of transformed
system of, 85–86
private versus single-payer,
75–81
research projects of
transformed system of,
88–89
strategies of transformed
system of, 87–88
transformation versus
reform, 83–93
values of transformed
system of, 86
health maintenance
organizations (HMOs),
11, 89
development of, 11–13
health savings accounts,
81–82
heart attack, 1,2, 27, 36, 65
Hileman, Bette, 41
Hippocrates, 45, 49, 50
Hippocratic Oath, 16, 47–
51, 55, 67
Hippocratic Oath, the, 47–
51
Hippocratic Oath, the, and
today's physicians, 48
HIV, 56
HIV/AIDS, 19
HMOs (*see* health
maintenance
organizations)
homeless population,
medical treatment of, 8,
19
homeopathy, 54 (*see also*
Complementary and
Alternative Medicine)
hypertension, 26, 32, 36, 56

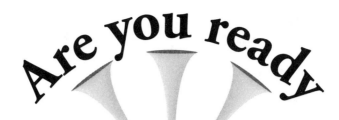

Are you ready

for real health reform?

THEN JOIN US!

National Alliance for Health Reform

Integrating Wellness and Prevention into U.S. Health Care

Together
WE CAN
and must
TRANSFORM
U.S. health care!

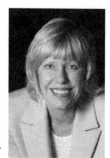

Dr. Mary Zennett, Founder
www.nationalallianceforhealthreform.org

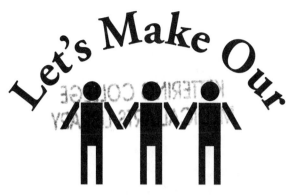

Let's Make Our

Voices Heard!

Join Dr Mary's health blog:
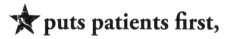
www.healthforusall.com

Introducing an innovative health care model that:

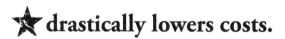

⭐ **puts patients first,**

⭐ **includes health, wellness and prevention; and**

⭐ **drastically lowers costs.**

Provide your experience, your ideas, your hopes for the future of U.S. health care

We want to hear from you!